Health and Social Care: Knowledge and Skills

Communication and Interpersonal Skills

D0569629

Health and Social Care: Knowledge and Skills

Communication and Interpersonal Skills

Elaine Donnelly and Lindsey Neville

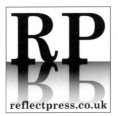

reflectpress.co.uk

The right of Elaine Donnelly and Lindsey Neville to be identified as authors of this work has been asserted by them in accordance with the Copyright, Designs and Patents Act 1988.

First published in 2008

ISBN: 978 1 906052 06 5

British Library Cataloguing in Publication Data
A catalogue record for this book is available from the British Library

Production project management by Deer Park Productions, Tavistock, Devon

Typeset by Pantek Arts Ltd, Maidstone, Kent

Cover design by Oxmed

Printed and bound by Cromwell Press Ltd, Trowbridge, Wiltshire

www.reflectpress.co.uk

Published by Reflect Press Ltd
11 Attwyll Avenue
Exeter
Devon
EX2 5HN
UK
Tel: 01392 204400

Contents

HEALTH AND SOCIAL CARE SERIES

Series Editors: Sue Cuthbert, Jan Quallington and Elaine Donnelly – all at the University of Worcester

This series of textbooks is aimed at students on Health and Social Care Foundation Degree programmes in FE and HE institutions. However, the books also provide short introductions to key topics for Common Foundation Programme modules and will be suitable for first-year undergraduate courses in a variety of Health and Social Care subject areas. Books in the series will also be useful for those returning to practice and for overseas nursing students. The series includes three types of textbook:

Knowledge and Skills books;

Theory and Practice books;

Specialist books that cover specific professions, topics and issues.

All titles in the series will address the common elements articulated in relevant sector skill frameworks such as, for example, Skills for Care, Skills for Health, the NHS Knowledge and Skills Framework and the Code of Practice for Social Care Workers.

OTHER TITLES IN THE SERIES INCLUDE:

An Introduction to the Principles and Practice of Care by Peter Unwin
ISBN: 978 1 906052 03 4 (publication due summer 2008)

Understanding Research and Evidence-based Practice by Bruce Lindsay
ISBN: 978 1 906052 01 0 (in print)

Values for Care Practice by Sue Cuthbert and Jan Quallington
ISBN: 978 1 906052 05 8 (in print)

Safe and Clean Care: Infection Prevention and Control for Health and Social Care Students by Tina Tilmouth with Simon Tilmouth
ISBN: 978 1 906052 08 9 (publication due summer 2008)

Work-based Learning and Practice Placement: A Textbook for Health and Social Care Edited by Graham Brotherton and Steven Parker
ISBN: 978 1 906052 12 6 (publication due summer 2008)

Essential Study Skills for Health and Social Care Edited by Marjorie Lloyd and Peggy Murphy
ISBN: 978 1 906052 14 0 (publication due summer 2008)

Visit **www.reflectpress.co.uk** for more details on these titles.

Introduction

HELLO AND WELCOME TO THIS BOOK

When people communicate with each other it is normal protocol to say hello and acknowledge the other person. The writing team would therefore like to say 'hello' to you and 'thank you for choosing this book'.

When you select any academic text to read it is our experience that the first thing you do is read the title and see how it relates to what you are studying. It's likely that you will then have a look at the preface, scan the chapter headings and check the summary detail. You then take the next step and read the first few lines of the introduction and it is here that you will make a decision as to whether or not it is the book for you.

WHO IS THIS BOOK FOR?

This book is primarily written to support students undertaking study in any field of health and social care. You may be studying single modules aimed at developing your communication and interpersonal skills or you may be studying a full course for health and social care practitioners like, for example, a Foundation Degree in Health and Social Care, a Diploma or Degree course in Nursing and Midwifery, a course in Social Work or, perhaps, a course designed for practitioners working in the Hospital and Emergency Care Services. Regardless of which programme of study you are undertaking, this book is written to provide you with a valuable introduction to the fascinating field of Interpersonal and Communication Skills and it will help you to meet the learning outcomes of your course.

WHAT DOES THE BOOK COVER?

Like many books in any subject it begins by offering definitions, and then explores the meaning of what it is to be a skilled communicator. We explore simple everyday issues such as courtesy and protocols and what can happen when we forget to apply these in practice. The writing team recognises that personal review and reflection can act as a powerful tool in the process of learning and you will be encouraged to reflect on a series of situations and then project the principles learned through these reflections onto your own working experience.

As the book develops you will be introduced to a variety of counselling practices and a broad range of helping skills with useful direction to further reading. As an overview of many things, the book seeks to provide a snapshot of some of the key theories and practices that surround working with people. These provide the reader with an excellent basis from which to start their study in learning and developing effective interpersonal and communication skills. Where possible we have provided details of relevant online resources, taking care to include those aspects that relate to the nature of the work that you do and recommending only *bona fide* websites for downloads.

When we first talked about writing this book we were very excited. It represented the perfect book to support our teaching. We envisaged that our readers would all be students new to the areas of study that surround health and social care and that they would be involved in working across a broad range of health and social care facilities and with a broad mix of people. The authors, are all involved in the teaching of communication and interpersonal skills, have developed an introductory text that explores communication as a 'skilled behaviour' for students working with people and is based on real teaching and learning activities that have been tried and tested in the classroom.

The book itself does not profess to be the definitive text – it is far too small to be that – but what it does do is present and explore some of the key issues and theories that surround effective communication. It explores what happens when communication goes wrong and outlines some possible solutions that you can put in place to limit the consequences of poor communication and to develop more successful communication systems. Good communication is the key to effective care and we hope that you enjoy developing and practising the skills presented here.

Happy studying.

Elaine Donnelly

AUTHOR BIOGRAPHIES

Elaine Donnelly

Elaine Donnelly is a Senior Lecturer in Health, Social Care and Psychology at the University of Worcester. Much of her teaching is within the field of nursing and she previously worked as a mental health nurse in a variety of mental health facilities including elderly care, acute psychiatry and the community. As a registered mental health nurse she has always been interested in what makes people behave as they do. Her first degree was in Psychology and she then undertook a Master of Science degree in Health and Social Care. Her research and teaching interests include communication and interpersonal skills, supporting student learning, psychology, psychological development, caring for dying people and their families and supporting the bereaved. As a teacher she has a facilitative style in the classroom, encouraging students to learn through their experience, from each other and through the process of reflection. This is her first venture in writing for publication and she has written the text in a similar way to her teaching style. Future texts are currently being considered.

Lindsey Neville

Lindsey Neville is a Senior Lecturer in Community and Social Welfare in the Institute of Health, Social Care and Psychology at the University of Worcester. She has qualified teacher status and has taught in primary, secondary, special, further and higher education settings. As a counsellor she has experience of working in education and in the voluntary sector with Relate. She is an accredited practitioner of both the British Association for Counselling and Psychotherapy and the Higher Education Academy.

Chapter 1

Introducing Key Concepts in Communication

Elaine Donnelly

Key themes

This chapter introduces the field of study and explores:

- the book in context;
- the importance of communication;
- moving towards a definition of communication;
- academic definitions;
- intra-personal communication and positive thinking;
- interpersonal communication.

Being able to communicate effectively is essential for any practitioner working with people. Good communication is central to providing good care and service. This book aims to launch you on an exploration of what it is to communicate effectively with others and the impact that good and bad communication has on the process of care.

THE BOOK IN CONTEXT

Chapter One provides an overview of what is to come. Like most academic texts the book begins with an examination of definitions and then introduces you to some of the incredibly complex phenomena that surround communication and interpersonal skills. Therefore, Chapter One serves as an introduction to many of the themes you will be studying later.

Chapter Two takes you on to focus on some of the key issues involved in communication with others. The mode and channel of communication play just as big a part in ensuring effective care as we do as people. It explores communication channels and offers an overview of two models of communication that will help you identify how communications take place and some of the influences on the communication process.

Chapter Three focuses on a psychological perspective of intra-personal communication and interpersonal skills. It introduces the work of Eric Berne and uses Transactional Analysis as a working theory to help you understand your own intra-personal communication processes and the communications that you have with others.

Chapter Four introduces you to the skills of counselling and explores the difference between counselling and counselling skills. It provides an overview of counselling perspectives, outlining the work of key theorists including Gerard Egan, Carl Rogers and John Heron. The chapter also touches on ethical and boundary issues in the counselling process and explores service user perspectives.

Chapter Five places these counselling skills in the context of 'helping relationships'. It explores ethical dilemmas, self disclosure, self care and development, the concept of transference and how to refer someone to formal counselling services.

Chapter Six serves to tie the book together by offering scenarios and case examples of communication processes. The chapter invites you to engage in some problem-solving activities by applying some of the principles that you will have learned by studying this book. This includes dealing with difficult people, being assertive, communication in teams, barriers to communication and getting your message across in the most effective way.

STUDYING WITH THIS BOOK

As you read through each chapter you will be invited to supplement your reading with a variety of activities. There is a number of different types of activity in this book.

Reading activities

Reading activities may involve you looking for and accessing a specific document or text relevant to your place of work or subject area of study. If the reading activity requires you to access detail from the internet we will provide an online web address. We may also encourage you to follow links provided via that address but, again, this is subject to your area of interest. We recognise that some of your supplementary study will be very specific to the area in which you work and the nature of the people you will be working with. To meet your needs we have, where possible, provided alternative online web addresses for you to select from.

Reflections

Reflecting on what you already know or have had experience of can be a powerful tool in helping you identify what you did and why you did something in a given situation. Reflection on your actions and reflection during your actions can help you to integrate new learning and enable you to become a more effective person. Reflective activities may also involve you being asked to imagine something relevant to the topic and to work your way through the same as if it were a real event.

Jasper (2003), in her book *Beginning Reflective Practice*, explores the concept of reflective practice in nursing and health care. Where we refer to important supplementary reading we will provide a full reference at the end of each chapter. Where possible we will recommend a variety of texts to provide you with an element of choice in what you read. For example, Johns (2004) *Becoming a Reflective Practitioner* is another useful text exploring the concept of reflection in practice. It is important that you understand and appreciate the impact that reflection can have on your learning.

Writing activities

For writing activities it would be helpful to have a pen and paper to hand to jot down notes or make lists to refer back to at a later point. Writing activities may also be involved in reading and reflecting activities. Some of the activities detailed above may invite you to share your thoughts and ideas with other people and have discussions about key elements of the subject being studied.

Whatever activity is suggested it is completely up to you as to how you study that particular concept. The text and information on these pages will come alive only when you interact with them. So, wecome to this book and enjoy your study of Communication and Interpersonal Skills.

THE IMPORTANCE OF GOOD COMMUNICATION

At the very heart of effective care, regardless of whether you are working in a professional capacity or as a volunteer, you seek to 'help' others.

Effective communication is the key to delivering high-quality help and care, regardless of the setting you work, or wish to work, within. Effective communication is recognised as a core condition for all people who work in public service.

Reading activity

Find and read one of the following documents that are relevant to your field of work or study. As you read, make notes about how you think the document demonstrates how important good communication is.

If you are studying to work in any social setting that involves children and young people find and read the policy document *Every Child Matters: Common Core Skills and Knowledge for the Children's Workforce*. This is available online at **www.everychildmatters.gov.uk**

If you are studying to, or work within, any National Health Service (NHS) setting, find and read the policy document *The NHS Knowledge and Skills Framework*. This is available online at **www.dh.gov.uk/en/index.htm**

Now that you have read the document most relevant to your field of study have a look at the other document and compare the detail. You will find lots of other interesting links that may be useful later on within your studies.

You will have found that both documents have effective communication as their first 'core condition' of working with people.

> Communication is a key aspect of all jobs in the NHS. This dimension underpins all the other dimensions in the KSF.
>
> (Agenda for Change Project Team, 2004)

> Good communication is central to working with children, young people, their families and carers. It is a fundamental part of the Common Core.
>
> (Children's Workforce Unit, 2005)

Communication is central to everything we do in health and social care. If any of our communication skills are poor or deficient in some way and we are not able to put in place alternative strategies, or if we are negligent in communicating something that is important, in whatever format that communication takes place, the people we claim to care for will be disadvantaged and may suffer in consequence. Constantly reviewing, maintaining and improving your communication skills is a very important part of your work not just as a student but also as a professional/voluntary worker. Good communication is not always easy so it is important for you to know a little about the basics of good communication to aid your reflections and study of how to improve your communication/interpersonal skills.

TOWARDS A DEFINITION OF COMMUNICATION

There are more than 1,000 definitions of communication in the *Oxford English Dictionary*. So where should we begin? Before pinning it down to specific definitions, let's begin by looking at what we understand, within the broader context, communication to be.

Writing activity

1. Jot down your own understanding of what the term 'communication' means.
2. Based on what you have jotted down, try to work those ideas into a working definition.

Creating a succinct definition that takes into account everything you have noted is an incredibly difficult thing to do and you could try to compare your notes with what your fellow students have written. Are there any comparisons to be made or are your definitions completely different?

My definition of communication

My initial list of what the term 'communication' means was very long. It is what this whole book is all about but, when I came to determine my own definition, my thoughts immediately focused on the notion that communication is about any interaction we have with others. This seemed nice and simple on the surface but as I started to tease the definition out I found several issues that needed to be worked through. The use of the word 'any' creates difficulty for me in exploring what I want to focus on and the use of the word 'others' over-complicates things too.

'Others' could be animals or other living things. I have been known to share my innermost thoughts with my cat (thank goodness he cannot repeat these to other people) and I have been seen talking to plants and vegetables in the garden. At the time of writing I am talking to my computer, not that it ever responds and perhaps that is the key. I decided to keep my definition simple and, in the context of this book, I define it to be any interaction that takes place between people.

Even though I have tried to keep it simple my definition is still very complicated. Our interactions don't take place just face to face, they take place on many different levels and we use a variety of different methods and many modes of delivery in getting our message across. So, the rider to my definition is that 'communication' is a very difficult term to pin down to one simple statement. When studying definitions of communication it is important to remember that definitions reflect the interest and background of the person making the definition, and may also reflect their perceptions and experiences, so, therefore, their definition is not necessarily true in every context.

How do we communicate?

So my next thoughts turn to the question of how we communicate. I have no doubt that you have considered this in your response to the writing activity. Communication can be anything from a personal text message from a friend, to a public advertisement on the side of a bus. It might be as simple as a smile or something technically complicated as a piece of software for a computer. Thinking about methods and modes and channels of communication is an important aspect of understanding what we mean by communication and this is explored further in Chapter Two.

When we come to study communication it quickly becomes clear just how complex a phenomenon it is, even though we all engage in it from the minute that we are conceived (if not before). On a personal level we communicate with the world around by the things that we say, the way that we say them, and the things that we do and the way that do them. It can be the clothes we wear, how we style our hair, the way we walk, the way we talk, the way we behave, and how we demonstrate our attitude to life. Communication is all of these things and much more.

Communication, values and wellbeing

Communication affects the way we feel about ourselves as well as the way we feel about others. According to Littlejohn and Foss (2005), how we communicate is associated with 'personal values', with our 'culture' and how we 'value others' as well as ourselves. We live in a multicultural society and we cannot just consider how we communicate (meaning ourselves within our own cultural group) – we must consider others and how they communicate too. *The NHS Knowledge Skills Framework* that you read earlier makes it quite clear that Communication (Core Dimension 1) is very closely linked with Equality and Diversity (Core Dimension 6). *The Common Core Skills and Knowledge* in *Every Child Matters* also makes it clear that communication is closely linked with ethical practice and respect for ourselves and others.

Psychologists study communication and have argued that at every age and stage of our lives communication is fundamental to our very being. We all have different levels at which we feel comfortable communicating but we all need to do so to keep us well and functioning (West and Turner, 2007). According to Bowlby (1969) and Crowley and Hunter (2005), in situations where human beings are isolated and consequently forced into non-communication, their mental and physical health deteriorate. In tiny babies non-communication can lead to very severe consequences and be life threatening (Bowlby, 1969).

I am confident that as a result of the writing activity above you are now aware of just how big a subject communication is and, as our main focus is interpersonal skills and communicating with others, perhaps you are now able to summarise this discussion and, as a result, would like to review your own definition before moving on to look at the definitions of others.

Definitions in academic study

In academic study it is always more useful to explore subject-specific definitions or, at least, definitions written by scholars within a particular discipline. Take the following definition, for example. Wood (2004) defines communication as 'a process in which individuals interact with and through symbols to create and interpret meaning'. On the surface this could be viewed simply as a collection of words but there are many levels in which you can explore this definition. Let us look at those words and how Wood explains her perceptions and understanding of what communication is. The definition uses the word 'process', which is commonly understood to be a series of actions or activities that produce something. The word 'individuals' suggests not just communicating with oneself but also with others. So communication, according to this definition, is about taking part or sharing actions with another person or with a group of people.

Symbols

Wood (2004) suggests that we use 'symbols' in our communication with ourselves and with others and that we 'create' and 'interpret meaning' through those symbols. This throws another interesting perspective into the definition. 'Symbols' are things that represent something else. They can be in the form of a material object, such as your country's national flag, or they could be in the form of a symbolic action such as a gesture.

Alongside this idea we need to put the notion that we then 'create' and 'interpret meanings' from such symbolism, either through a shared activity or via our own internal understanding. That seems relatively simple but the creation and interpretation of symbols can present us with all sorts of difficulty because symbols can be interpreted differently by different people and their use in communication can be a little precarious.

Reflection

1. Have in front of you a small piece of paper, approximately 2 inches by 3 inches (5cm by 7.5cm), and colour it in red. Paint, felt tip or crayon will do nicely. Look at that piece of red paper. Does it mean anything to you?

2. Now imagine yourself holding that small piece of red paper above your head in a busy supermarket. Would the action of holding up your art work mean anything to the people around you? How do you think people would react to you? How do you think you would feel?

It is more than likely that people would perceive you as a little 'odd' and, consequently, having had a little peek at you (we are all curious beings after all) the people around you would ignore you and get on with their shopping and perhaps you would be left feeling a little foolish.

Now imagine that you are a referee on a football pitch. That little piece of red paper, all of a sudden, takes on new meaning. It has a symbolic function. It is seen as a Red Card. The Red Card, according to our understanding of football, symbolises that one of the players is judged by the referee to be guilty of a serious misdemeanour and is to be sent off the pitch. If you were the referee it is likely that you wouldn't feel foolish in this situation at all; rather you would feel noticed, validated, powerful and in charge. Although, perhaps, my perceptions of what it is to be a referee are a little at odds with reality. But whose reality? This is an important issue. It seems that we all share common realities and understand symbols that are meaningful to us but each of us also has our own interpretations of the world and these interpretations are influenced by some of the factors that Littlejohn and Foss (2005) outline in relation to values, social groups and culture.

I am going to follow this through a little more as it raises important issues for us to understand. If we were observers of the football game, regardless of how big the stadium was or how many people were there, we would easily spot a small piece of red card in the hand of the man dressed in black, and we instantly recognise the meaning of the action and the symbolism of the card. Knowing the Red Card's function we will respond, but our response isn't always absolutely predictable, even if we all interpreted the symbolic action the same way. Our response to observing the Red Card will be in accordance with whether or not we support the referee's decision to give a Red Card. Our interpretation of the referee's action is likely to reflect where our support lies; is it someone on our own team who is being sent off or someone on the opposite side? Our response could be predicted by the colour of the scarf or rosette that we wear and/or by the end of the stadium at which we stand while the game is being played. However, our responses to symbols are not always this clear cut.

So, something as simple as a Red Card triggers all sorts of communications and interactions among people. We all see the same symbol and we all understand the meaning, but we interpret the referee's behaviour differently. Some of us may cheer ecstatically while others boo and hiss as loudly as possible and then there are those who would go on to discuss the ins and outs of the decision for ever (can you detect from my communication that I dislike post-mortems of football matches? How did you detect that?).

Reflection

1. Can you think of other examples of symbols and symbolic actions in everyday life and how we attribute meaning to them?

2. How does that attribution of meaning influence our behaviour?

3. What are the possible consequences of symbols and symbolic actions being misinterpreted by others?

I'm sure that you were able to think of many circumstances where symbols influence your behaviour. Road traffic signs are a good example of how a symbol can influence our behaviour. The speed camera sign always makes me check my speed and traffic signage uses simple symbols to convey a whole host of messages targeted at influencing our driving behaviour. Symbols can create unity and symbols can create tension. Symbolic acts have started wars, sparked revolution and changed lives, and whether those changes were good or bad is down to your interpretation of them.

The definition offered by Wood (2004) raises some essential issues in studying communication that I was not able to raise in my definition earlier. It is important that we stop and make the time to explore definitions and try to see the world as others perceive it to be. It will enrich our understanding and enable us to make more positive decisions about how we communicate. Communication is about who we are. It isn't a single one-off thing. It is a very complicated process and to assist you in understanding some of the complexities involved in communicating with yourself and with others I have broken it down into different areas for study. The first of these areas is intra-personal communication.

INTRA-PERSONAL COMMUNICATION

The way we communicate with others is known as interpersonal communication and we will look at that process later, but first we will look at this notion of intra-personal communication. Intra-personal communication can be described as a constant dialogue within ourselves (Cauchon, 1994). All of our communications are influenced by how we feel at the time and how we perceive ourselves to be. Intra-personal communication is a cognitive function in that it is about the things that we think but it is also plays a significant part in our emotions and how we understand the world to be and our place in it. As humans we self regulate our behaviour and how we self regulate and respond to our innermost feelings and thoughts has an impact on how we present ourselves to the world. Whatever we see, hear, smell or feel as part of that communication is

- evaluated by our brains based on past knowledge and experience;
- reviewed by our senses;
- and then evaluated again.

This inner process often continues even after the 'physical communication' has ended. An example of this is that of replaying a conversation time and time again in our heads, imagining the different responses that we, and the other people involved, could have made. We often imagine not just what might have been said, but the looks that might have been exchanged, the gestures that we might make, even the emotions we or the other person might feel. The outcome in our head may be completely different from the outcome that was achieved. Our memory of the event may be recalled by simple triggers such as a word, a smell, a sound or the feel of something that reminds us of the previous occasion. But memories are not always a reliable source of what actually happened; they merely represent our perceptions of the event at the time.

Memories are often built upon as we make our experiences meaningful to us and that is how stories evolve. Stories and personal narratives are very important in helping us make sense of our experience, and the telling of narrative is an important method of communicating with others, but it is that process of constructing narratives that leads us to have different perceptions of events from other people even though we may share the same experience.

Reflection

1. Look at a family photograph that is important to you. What do you recall about that time/the day the photo was taken?
2. How would those who were around you at that time recall that event? Is their perception the same as or different from yours?

It may be that you and others remember the day on which the photograph was taken but it is likely that your experiences of the day will be different from those of the other person. What influenced you on the day and your memory-recall reflects what was important to you at the time and how you felt but this may not be the same as the other person's experience. Individuals in families will often give different accounts of their childhood even though they were exposed to very similar experiences. What was really exciting for one is viewed as really scary by another and results in different feelings, different thoughts and different perspectives of events. Differences in experiences may be a major cause of friction within those family relationships.

As humans we not only consider and review the past but we also engage in thinking about conversations that we are going to have in the future. This is another example of intra-personal dialogue with ourselves. We all rehearse conversations. You only have to sit in traffic and observe people in their cars, where there is an element of privacy, and there are many people having a conversation with themselves. Talking to oneself is a natural activity that we all engage in and thinking aloud often proves to be a really useful way of preparing for, or dealing with, a problem, although it can be the source of embarrassment when we are caught out by someone who overhears. We often then try to cover up our conversation with ourselves by humming or singing or pretending that we were not talking to ourselves at all, unless we are actors, in which case we can comfortably say we are rehearsing our lines.

In a nutshell, intra-personal communication involves internal dialogue with oneself. It may involve rehearsal and even the analysis of personal thoughts, dreams, fantasies and perceptions. As we experience those inner thoughts we also experience feelings which in turn affect how we behave when communicating or making contact with someone else.

Reflection

You find a purse/wallet under your table in a restaurant. What would you do?

What you choose to do is directly influenced by previous experience, by the teachings of your care givers (usually parents and teachers but others may be included here) and by what you have learned. This reflective activity may include you reviewing your moral codes of behaviour and your values. Is it 'finders keepers' or is it sympathy with the person who has lost the purse/wallet? Perhaps this has happened to you. Losing your purse or wallet isn't just about losing money – it often involves losing other important items that you keep within it. Do you remember how you felt?

Maybe you would immediately, almost without thought, raise the attention of the waiter and hand the purse/wallet over to the establishment for safe keeping. Perhaps you would hesitate before taking action. Maybe you don't like the look of the waiter – does he seem honest to you? In this circumstance you might engage in an internal conversation with yourself where you listen to the 'little voice in your head' (sometimes referred to as your conscience) and take action to find the owner yourself. You can check inside the purse/wallet for some form of identification or contact details. If you found limited money, a bus pass, a prescription for anti-depressants and a faded photograph of a young soldier perhaps you would be more likely to actively search for the owner than if you found lots of money, a first-class rail ticket, several Platinum credit cards and a membership card to an exclusive health/golf club? Whatever your decision, intrapersonal communication has a big effect on your behaviour. You can explore that further by changing some aspect of the scenario. What if you found the purse/wallet in the place where you work?

Negative thinking

Most of us think before we speak, even though we may not be aware of it at the time. The thoughts that precede action are often automatic thoughts that are well rehearsed. For some people automatic thoughts are self deprecating and, when this is extreme, it may lead to a cognitive/affective disorder such as depression or a person becoming obsessive about certain aspects of their lives. We will look at this further in Chapter Three when we use Transactional Analysis (TA) to explore internal dialogue, but there are other theories that can help us understand how thinking influences feelings and vice versa. Cognitive Behavioural Therapy (CBT) as established by Arron Beck (1989) seeks to help the person change how they think and feel about themselves. Abramowitz (2001) suggests that CBT is a really effective technique that can be used in almost any setting. Developing such a skill may prove to be of interest to you as you progress through your studies but that detail is not explored any further here other than to give you these references for further reading.

What is evidenced in those texts and similar writings is that how we think and feel about ourselves impacts on our behaviour and consequently on how we communicate with the world. The more positive we are in our thoughts and perceptions of the world and ourselves, the more likely it is that we are more positive in our communications with others. Goleman (1996), in his book *Emotional Intelligence*, describes what he terms the 'Master Aptitude' in which he explores how personal narrative and self talk influence us as human beings. If we believe we can do a thing the likelihood is that we can. For Goleman 'hope' and 'optimism' are our great motivational forces and it is positive thinking that makes all the difference to our mood, our emotional sense of self, how we communicate, and our success.

For example, if we believe ourselves to be hopeless at something like speaking French we try to avoid speaking it and rely on others to communicate for us if the need arises. We would hold ourselves back from the conversation and push others ahead to do the talking. The thoughts that may go through your head in that situation may include, 'I'm not good enough, my French teacher was always telling me my accent was atrocious, I will make a total fool of myself, best to leave it up to the others'. The consequences of holding back may then be perceived by others involved in that communication as our being lazy, shy or just plain ignorant. It all depends upon the other person's interpretation of our avoidance behaviour. They may then throw us a look that results in us feeling even more inadequate and more negative about the situation and ourselves. It reinforces our negative thinking about how hopeless we actually are and it can tap into previous memories and similar experiences when we felt like this. Inevitably this leads to more negative thinking, which impacts further on our behaviour and may make us even more resistant to speaking French. We develop patterns of behaviour that initially seek to protect us but often result in an over-reaction to a given situation. I leave you to think of the consequences.

This example used speaking another language but you can replace speaking French with doing maths or something that you feel you are not good at and the result is likely to be avoidance behaviour and negative thinking. Negative thinking often leads to poor performance which, in turn, is reinforced by ourselves and maybe even by others.

Reflection

1. Can you think of another personal event or issue that you have that leads to this downward spiral of negative thinking?

2. How does that impact on your behaviour?

3. What is the outcome of that behaviour on you and on others?

4. Can you think of ways in which you could change the outcome?

5. What do you imagine the result would be?

We've all been in situations that we know we could have handled differently and where the outcome could have been more beneficial to all concerned if only we had gone about it in a different way. One of the techniques many people use to counteract these negative responses is self talk. Using key words like 'steady', 'focus', 'stay with the moment', 'don't panic', 'think', 'breathe in slowly', 'take your time' are tools we often use to help us regulate our thoughts and behaviour. Changing the dialogue in your head is a good technique to avoid falling into patterns of behaviour and using positive thinking can cancel out the negative thoughts.

Positive thinking

The power of positive thinking should never be underestimated. Positive thinking can enhance our performance enormously. Positive thinkers engage in positive internal dialogue that reinforces and affirms their competence and their ability to do well. We occasionally get to see or read about famous people and what they do to 'psych themselves up' before going on stage. That's the power of positive thinking – it changes our mind-set and results in different behaviour. If we think positively we will feel positive and it is then more than likely that we will act in a different way.

You may have techniques to get yourself through tricky situations. Warming up by clapping, thinking or even thinking the words 'come on, I can do this' are all examples of positive internal dialogue. As you 'warm up' you may even verbalise or portray some of those warming-up actions and share them with others. The result may be that you gain their support which, in turn, has the potential to improve your performance or at least your mind-set. In a situation where everyone is backing you, urging you on, clapping and offering their support you are encouraged and your behaviour will be changed or enhanced in some way.

The positive person is generally more successful in their relationships and in life. Developing the skill of reflection and examining your own internal thoughts and patterns of behaviour can help enormously. We will look at how that internal dialogue can be challenged and changed in Chapter Two.

INTERPERSONAL SKILLS

Being competent in interpersonal communication is crucial for successful living and all communication theorists define interpersonal skills in a similar way. A skill is something that is seen as a motor activity that can be practised, developed and refined until perfection is achieved (Hargie 1991). However, interpersonal skills are far more complex than that and involve a whole host of factors.

Writing activity

1. Make a list of all the interpersonal skills you know. The list may be divided into those interpersonal skills you have and those skills you wish to develop in the future and may be divided further into subcategories if you wish. It's your perception and understanding of what constitutes an interpersonal skill that counts.

2. Now discuss your list with another person who you feel will be able to give you valuable feedback about your skills and, perhaps, add to the overall list.

3. Write down your thoughts on how and where we develop interpersonal skills and follow this through by using an example of your own.

No doubt your list is a long one detailing all sorts of things ranging from assertiveness to values, attitude to understanding, empathy to questioning. You may have included clusters of communication skills such as verbal and non-verbal behaviours and it is likely that you have used some of the previous detail in responding to the second question.

If you have discussed this with someone you should have an insight into how skilled a person you already are and gained some insight into how you have developed those skills. When I teach this subject in the classroom my students are very clear about how and where they developed their interpersonal skills and it is likely that your response is similar. Interpersonal skills are learned. They are learned through observation and practice, they are a result of previous experience and intra-personal evaluation. We begin to learn interpersonal skills during childhood and we can continue to develop them throughout our lives.

Interpersonal skills are culture-bound, age-related and often gender-specific. They reflect the sort of person we are. We often use interpersonal skills without thinking as they are so ingrained within our behaviour. Through reflection and detailed analysis, alongside a desire to learn, we can develop and refine those skills. Becoming more competent at human communication will enable you to become more competent in your role of helping others.

Definitions of interpersonal skills

Because the factors involved are so many it is difficult to find a succinct academic definition that addresses all of these issues. Burnard (1989) commented that 'what constitutes interpersonal skills is vast', and he goes on to suggest that 'personal qualities are a necessary pre-requisite for effective interpersonal relationships'. It is likely that you either work, or you are going to work, in areas that require you to have effective personal relationships with those whom you work with. It is therefore essential that you develop and demonstrate these qualities. The personal qualities that Burnard (1989) alludes to are based on those of Carl Rogers (1967) and include 'warmth and genuineness, empathic understanding and unconditional positive regard'. As Burnard states, 'it is these qualities that form the basis and the bedrock of all effective human relationships'. These qualities underpin helping relationships and are further discussed in Chapters Four and Five where helping and counselling skills are explored.

This chapter has introduced definitions of communication, made the link between communication skills, intra-personal skills and interpersonal skills and briefly mentioned counselling skills. The next chapter will explore communications in practice and, in particular, it will focus on methods of communication.

Chapter 2

Exploring Communication in Practice

Elaine Donnelly and Tim Johnson

Key themes

This chapter explores

- modes of communication;
- communicating with people who use health and social care services;
- choosing your approach in communicating with others;
- studying communications theory;
- frameworks of communication;
- two models of communication;
- channels of communication.

The first chapter of this book gave a broad perspective on how we communicate. Much of the 'helping' communication in the health and social care field takes place on a face-to-face basis but a great deal of communication also takes place using alternative means. This chapter explores some of the many modes and channels of communication and introduces two models of communication to enable you to become more aware of communication processes.

MODES OF COMMUNICATION

Messages are communicated in many different ways. New methods of transmission and new channels of communication are developing at an incredibly rapid pace as we progress into the digital age. Over the last 50 years the developments in technology have had a massive impact on how we communicate with each other. We can connect with someone on the other side of the world with a click of a mouse and with someone on the moon at the flick of a switch. Information technology has changed the world we live in more than any other technical phenomenon.

Taylor (2003) discusses the use of Information Communications Technology (ICT) with particular reference to its use when studying. When studying in any field of health and social care you will find that ICT is playing an increasingly important role in how we deliver, record and monitor care. As practitioners in whatever field you work, you have a responsibility to develop and update your skills accordingly.

Writing activity

1. Think of all the different ways your grandparents and your great-grandparents may have communicated with each other and the rest of the world as young people, and draw up a list of these.
2. If you have the opportunity, speak with a person aged 80 years plus and see if they can confirm the ways you have identified. They may be able to add to your list with some very interesting examples of means of communication. No doubt some of their methods were quite innovative, particularly if they involved speaking with boyfriends and girlfriends without their parents being aware and, of course, communicating during the war years.

Perhaps your list will have included some of the following:

- face-to-face, person-to-person conversation;
- whistling, singing and calling out loud;
- telephone, via the operator of course;
- writing, including letters, postcards, poetry and song;
- handwritten records and ledgers and typed correspondence;
- telegraphy, telegrams and couriers;
- sign language and ticktack, and secret gestures;
- secret codes and messaging banners, flags and semaphore;
- flickering lights, and opening and shutting curtains;
- pigeon post and go-betweens, flares and other pyrotechnics;
- radio, television and cinema.

These are only the examples we could come up with but no doubt there are many more.

Writing activity

1. Cover the next section of text and extend your list to include all modes and methods of communication that you have seen or taken part in, either in your personal life or in your experience of work. It is likely to be quite long... Then compare what you have written with the list we have generated below.

- Text messaging, e.mail and MSN messenger.
- Telephone (land line) and mobile phone.
- Blue tooth, BLOG and podcasts.
- Computers, laptops and Blackberry.
- Web pages, MMS messages, U Tube and MySpace.
- Music, rap and Bebo.
- Satellite communications such as GPS and Sat Nav.
- Electronic records and online forms.
- Care documentation and care plans.
- Voice mail, pagers, bleeps and alarms.
- Radio waves, x-rays and scans.

This is by no means a comprehensive list and we are sure you can think of others. Channels of communication are developing all the time and this requires us to be engaged in learning and developing our skills in communication throughout our lives.

COMMUNICATING WITH PEOPLE WHO USE HEALTH AND SOCIAL CARE SERVICES

In health and social care services effective communication promotes the best possible care. It can safeguard you in the case of legal or disciplinary action and it empowers you to practise the highest possible standards of care. The way we communicate with people who use our service or facility also has a direct impact on how care is perceived and experienced. More complaints are made about practitioners whose communication skills are poor than about professional expertise (Gladwell, 2005). Patient Advice and Liaison Services (PALS) annual reports, which are all available on the web (at, for example, **www.eastern.nhs.uk**) regularly detail staff attitude and poor communication skills as the main area of complaint. We'll come back to this later.

Reflection

Think about the way health and social care providers communicate with people who use their services. It might be helpful to physically walk around your workplace and observe the means of communication used there, or walk around a service facility that is open to the public or one that you would use. Make a mental note of what you see around you and consider the essence of the communications you observed.

1. How would you describe these communications?
2. What form do they take and how do they make you feel?

To explore this further we are going to use our own experience of going to our local GP surgery/health centre as it is likely that all of you have visited your local facility. In an average GP surgery or health centre you will be able to observe and experience many different formats of communication, including most of the following.

- To get an appointment with anyone who works at the health centre it is likely that you will have to telephone first. This may involve you being placed in a telephone queue, pressing appropriate telephone buttons and it may take a little time.
- You will have to converse with a receptionist (fingers crossed that he or she can understand your use of verbal language, accent, dialect, etc.) and negotiate your appointment in relation to the urgency of your request and the person whom you would most like to see or deal with.
- When you arrive at the centre there are lots of directional instructions regarding where you can park (your car or your pushchair), where you should enter the building and that 'children should be under supervision'.
- As you enter the building there will be lots of health care/promotional posters on the walls. These are usually instructional and involve detail about the dangers or benefits of several everyday activities such as smoking, drinking alcohol and drug abuse. Magazines and health information leaflets are also likely to be available for your perusal.
- A zero tolerance poster stating that aggressive or rude behaviour will not be tolerated is now common in health centres, as are signs that say all mobile telephones should be turned off. There will also be some signage about health and safety, in particular about fire assembly points, and signs directing you to toilet facilities.
- There may be a television screen that flashes up messages regarding services available at the health centre and promoting flu jabs, etc. and it may tell you how many people missed their appointment last week.
- There may be a touch screen on which you can key in your arrival and confirm your appointment and there may be signage telling you that if you are waiting to see a certain person they have a trainee working with them and that, with your permission, the interview will be recorded.
- There may be a bell or light system indicating when you should enter the consulting room or you may have to wait on the nod of the receptionist. The person that you have come to see may shout your name down the corridor or even come and collect you from the waiting area.
- You might find yourself offered the opportunity to complete a questionnaire about your experience and satisfaction with the service.
- Lots of this detail will be presented in different languages that represent those spoken in the local community.

All this and you don't feel very well ... The health centre used in this example is a newly-built facility. It was bright and freshly painted and the communications were all up-to-date. The receptionists were most helpful and look very smart in their new uniforms and we were delighted to find that e.mail requests for repeat prescriptions are accepted and that there is a prescription collection and delivery service offered via local pharmacies. Our feelings about this health centre were generally positive, although the amount of instructional material was a little overwhelming (but it did give us something to do while waiting for the appointment). Some of the messages displayed will have an impact on our immediate behaviour so, for example, if your mobile phone rings you are likely to turn it off quickly, but many of the messages are part of a much bigger campaign to get health messages across to the general public and on their own they are often ignored.

However, sadly, we do have experiences of visiting other health care organisations where the facilities are lacking, the receptionists are rude, the décor is drab, toilets are dirty and information available is not up-to-date. All of this has an impact upon us as users of the service and we are more likely to be unhappy about our consultation even before we meet the professional we have booked to see.

Reflection

The environment plays a big part in how we view services available to us. When you go back to your place of work or when you start work in a new environment what does the setting say about your service?

1. If your perception is negative, how do you think service users view the service?
2. How does the environment impact on the people who work there and the people who use the service?

We leave that with you to decide. You might feel it appropriate to take action and discuss issues with your supervisor.

Writing activity

Good customer care has to be part of everyone's agenda in raising standards and ensuring quality, but how well do we do when inviting a person or a family to use our services? If you were inviting a group of people, who are important contacts for a future project, to your house for dinner, what measures would you take to make sure they can find where you live and that dinner is a success?

1. Draw up a list of things to do.
2. Talk your list through with a colleague or friend and compare your list with what they would do.

Here's what we would do. First, we would check that our guests knew how to get to our houses. We both agreed that we would have checked at the point of invitation if they had any food preferences – there is nothing worse than serving goulash to vegetarians. We both commented that we would think very carefully about what food and drink to serve and it is more than likely that we would clean the house, focusing special attention on the bathroom and those areas of the house we would be using. We would also think about what clothes to wear and probably go to some trouble in terms of our own presentation and, finally, we would consider putting the cat out and covering up the pet lizard and stick insects just in case our guests found them distasteful. In summary, we both agreed that anticipating guest-needs is an important part of our preparation and we had awful stories to tell when we had not been quite on the ball. Did you consider similar things?

When we invite people into our homes we generally like to make a good impression, but is that social courtesy extended to the place where we work and to the people to whom we provide a service? Our experience says not. There have been occasions when both of us have used services and been really impressed with how the service was managed and how we as individuals were dealt with. However, there are still lots of service facilities that do not meet with basic quality standards and fail to achieve benchmarks set by their own organisational quality assurance processes.

At the time of writing there is a great deal of media coverage regarding how dirty our hospitals are and there are many debates about how best to overcome the problem. While recognising that some of the problems are down to the age and infrastructure of the building, it is suggested that a great deal of dirtiness and, consequently, the spread of hospital-acquired infections, is down to poor management and practice (**www.bbcnews.co.uk**). Solutions that have been put forward to combat these problems include strengthening communication systems, advertising hand-washing protocols using posters that encourage patients and their relatives to speak out if their practitioner doesn't wash their hands and even, in one NHS Trust, the use of hospital radio announcements reminding everyone to 'wash their hands'. Poor communication processes are often found to be at the heart of a problem and improving communications its solution.

CHOOSING YOUR APPROACH WHEN COMMUNICATING WITH OTHERS

When communicating directly with people, you first need to choose the mode or the approach that you are going to use and, to be effective in getting your message across, you need to consider some key issues.

Reflection

Imagine yourself in the workplace and being involved in communicating with a person or several people about future plans. What methods or channels of communication might you consider before engaging in that communication? Share your considerations with a colleague.

Your reflection and discussions may have involved you considering some of the following.

- Will the communication be face-to-face, written or using technology?
- Will you use letters, pictures or leaflets in the communication to help clarify what it is you are communicating?
- How much control do you have over the environment and how much control do you have over the timing of the communication?
- How many people are you communicating with and what level of understanding do they have?
- Are there any language or disability issues to consider?
- Do you want people to respond to you and, if so, how do you want them to respond to you?
- Do you want people to have the opportunity to ask questions and how much information do you need to get back from them?
- How detailed should the communication be and how important is this communication at this point?

When communicating with people in the workplace it is important that we think carefully about the channel of communication we use so that we can make sure we pick the most effective method for them. People are individuals and what is satisfactory for one may be completely inappropriate for another. If you are working with families you may have to use several channels of communication, and to target individual members. A leaflet and a quick explanation may suffice in some circumstances but, in others, we need to employ a wide range of interpersonal and communication skills to ensure that what we do is effective for everyone concerned.

STUDYING COMMUNICATIONS THEORY

Studying communications theory can help us to understand how communication works and help us to determine the most effective communication channel to use. Knowing how communication works, we can then understand how, why and where communication goes wrong. When communication goes wrong in health and/or social care settings the consequences can be far-reaching. People and families can be misjudged, errors in decision-making can be made and care may be seriously compromised, leaving you and the people you care for at risk.

If we can identify how communication takes place and understand its process we can develop strategies to ensure that communication is effective and meets the needs of all concerned. To help you understand communication we are first going to look at the key frameworks within which the theories and models of communication are set.

Frameworks of communication

There are four main frameworks for theories of communication. These are:

- **Mechanistic** – this framework was originally used by people working on radio and telephone communications and incorporates a transmission model of communication.
- **Psychological** – this framework concentrates far more on how we feel during a communication and our emotional responses.
- **Social Constructionist** – this framework is concerned with how we all construct different realities from the same experiences. The Symbolic Interaction Theory that we will be looking at is included in this framework.
- **Systemic** – this framework concentrates on the way that communication is part of a whole system and how, within that system, each part of the communication is repeatedly re-examined and reworked.

We are going to look at two models of communication within these frameworks. The first is a Transmission Model. This type of model is included in the Mechanistic Framework and is said to be linear in its process. It is a simple straightforward model that is easy to understand and can be very useful in helping analyse communication processes between people and organisations.

The second model we will look at is a Transactional Model that combines principles from the Psychological, Social Constructionist and Systemic frameworks. The Transactional Model is slightly more complicated than the Mechanistic one and further explores the experience of shared meanings in our communications with others that we discussed in Chapter One. We will then follow an example of a Transactional Model in practice by exploring the psychotherapeutic theory of Transactional Analysis in Chapter Three.

The Shannon and Weaver Transmission Model

One of the earliest, most basic and well-known communication models is that of Shannon and Weaver (1949). Their model is sometimes referred to as the 'Mother of Communication Models' and it provides a good starting point for anyone studying communication theory.

As you can see in Figure 1, the arrows that show transmission from the Information Source to the Destination point in only one direction, reflecting the belief that messages flow in only one direction at any given time. It is therefore a linear process.

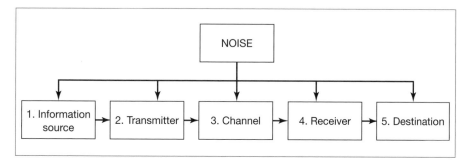

Figure 1 The Shannon and Weaver Transmission Model

The Shannon and Weaver model consists of five parts and what they term 'Noise'. In a face-to-face communication

1. the information would be the idea that you had in your head;
2. the transmitter would be you sending the message;
3. the channel would be your voice as you speak the idea;
4. the receiver would be the ear of the person to whom you are talking;
5. the destination would be the intended person's head.

Noise, as you can see, can occur at any point within that communication process, and can prevent the original thought or idea reaching its destination intact and as intended. Noise can be anything. Noise might be

- physical, i.e. what we commonly call noise, a loud sound (physical noise);
- psychological, i.e. an emotion such as anxiety or a strongly-held point of view or a cultural barrier (psychological noise);
- semantic, i.e. a language or representation problem (semantic noise);
- physiological, i.e. deafness, blindness or pain (physiological noise).

Noise can interrupt the communication at any stage.

Reflection

1. Imagine yourself in a busy work area. What sorts of noise do you think might stop your message getting through to another person?
   - Are people or machines making a 'noise'?
   - Is the other person in an emotional state, are they flustered, worried, angry or even frightened?
   - Is their perception of the situation different from yours?
   - Do they understand the language you are using?
   - Do they have a particular communication problem?

2. Make a list of some of the common things that you think would cause 'noise' and interfere with communications in your place of work, and discuss your experiences with a colleague. It might help if you list the noises under the headings offered. You'll be surprised at what constitutes 'noise', particularly when you explore the psychological aspect.

If your message is not getting across, this simple model gives you the opportunity to explore some of the reasons why. Once the 'noise' is identified you can then try to eliminate or at least modify the 'noise' or message in some way. The possibilities are all subject to the nature of the 'noise' and may require you to do some strategic thinking and extra planning to ensure your message gets across. Can you think of any recent examples of 'noise' interfering with a message you wanted to convey? Now that you have been introduced to this model, can you think of tools or techniques that may have helped you overcome that noise at the time?

As teachers we experience 'noise' in the learning situation all the time, particularly in the large groups that we sometimes have to teach. We often hear colleagues say, 'I told the students yesterday, why don't they listen?' Our response is always the same. Telling someone something doesn't mean they have heard what you say and, using Shannon and Weaver's model, our approach is to identify the 'noise' that stopped the message getting across and to try other ways to make sure the message is delivered, heard and understood. Other methods to overcome noise in this example will often involve using alternative modes and channels of communication including announcements, notices, ICT, other people, good old repeating oneself, using humour to capture attention, jumping up and down or sometimes even whispering. These are all strategies that we use in the classroom. The strategies you use should be appropriate to the situation and to the person or people you are communicating with. Never believe that people have heard exactly what you meant to say without first checking their understanding and making sure the message reached its destination intact and as you intended it. Using such a simple strategy will help avoid all sorts of complications later on.

Julia Wood's Transactional Model

The other model of communication to be discussed here is a Transactional Model. Chapter 1 (pages 7–10) introduced the work of Julia Wood (2004) and explored her definition of communication. You will recall that communication is:

> A systemic process in which individuals interact with and through symbols to create and interpret meanings.
>
> (Wood, 2004)

That definition was then broken down into components for analysis, and part of the discussion in Chapter One explored the significance of symbols in our communication, how they impact upon our behaviour and how we create and interpret meanings through that process.

Wood (2004) offers the following diagram (Figure 2) to illustrate communications taking place between two people.

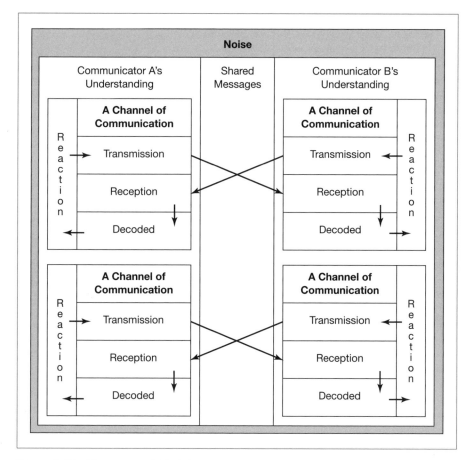

Figure 2 The Transactional Model

In this model you can see that communicator **A** transmits a message to communicator **B** who receives the message, decodes the message, has a reaction to the message and then responds to communicator **A**. Notice that the 'noise' surrounds the process and that 'shared messages' have a direct impact on the communication between the two.

This is a far more complex model of communication than Shannon and Weaver's which, you will recall, was linear in its process. In this model messages are being sent backwards and forwards all the time, not just in one direction but simultaneously. The Transactional Model focuses on how we interpret meaning and how meanings are shared within our communication with other people. When communication goes wrong it is often the result of meaning being misinterpreted. Meaning in communication is said to be negotiated between the people concerned. For example, if you use a word in one context with friends it will be interpreted in a particular way by that social group but, use the same word or communication with your teachers or parents, and the meaning is not shared on the same level. For example, the words 'wicked', ' whatever' and 'hot' come to mind, as we know our interpretations of these words are completely different from those of younger people. There are, no doubt, lots of other examples you can think of. Our language is constantly developing and has to accommodate new ways of living, new technologies and new ways of expressing feelings and thoughts. Social groups use a common language to communicate on a psychological and sociological level that isn't always instantly apparent to people on the outside of that group.

The language we use, our non-verbal behaviours and the symbols we include in our communications all play a powerful role in establishing and sharing meaning. It is important to remember that understanding something is a subjective experience. We construct meaning in social contexts and share a mutual awareness and often a mutual language that is culturally bound and age-related.

It is interesting to note that in an average face-to-face communication, 55 per cent of what is communicated is said to be communicated via body language, 38 per cent is communicated via voice tonality (sometimes included in what is called non-verbal vocalisations) and only 7 per cent of the communication relies on the actual words spoken (see Figure 3).

We all know that our words can be misunderstood, sometimes because we are using words that the other person does not understand. Sometimes the words are right but another part of our communication is misunderstood. The meaning that underlines our voice tonality, our body language and our words can all be misinterpreted. Cultural differences affect even simple gestures and because we communicate using symbols, social differences,

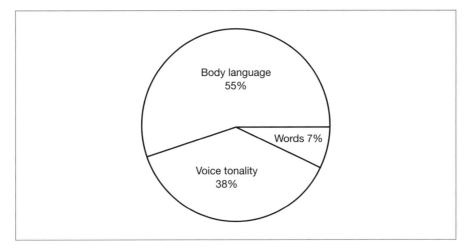

Figure 3 Communication Pie Chart

even within the same culture, can affect communication. Most of the symbols we use during communication are learned when we are young and, therefore, some communication is not just culturally specific, it can also be specific to a family because you learn your basic communication symbols from your family. For one person the symbolic meaning of an extended period of eye-to-eye contact might mean that you are interested in what they have to say, while for another it could mean that you are being aggressive or threatening towards them.

Non-verbal communication, just like speech, is also affected by gender and social status. The Transactional Model is a much better model of what really happens in face-to-face communication than the Shannon and Weaver model. The Transactional Model takes into consideration all the aspects of communication that we looked at in Chapter One. It is also a better basis for any new communication system you might consider creating to help the people you work with. What is it in the Transactional Model that makes it so much better at explaining what real-life communication is like? The answer lies in the channels of communication.

Channels of communication

In the Transactional Model multiple channels are being used. For example:

- facial expressions;
- body angle;
- posture;
- presentation;
- tone of voice;
- words;

South Essex College
Further & Higher Education, Southend Campus
Luker Road Southend-on-Sea Essex SS1 1ND
Tel: 01702 220400 Fax: 01702 432320
Minicom: 01702 220642

29

- word images;
- role portrayal.

If you refer back to Figure 2 you will see that not only are multiple channels being used but the arrows point both ways instead of in just one way. The person sending the message is at the same time receiving a message through the same channels. As each person receives a message they are simultaneously decoding it. They are using all their previous experiences and memories to sift through what they are receiving in order to give meaning to it. At the same time they are creating and sending their own message and there is still all that 'noise' going on around the communications being sent, received and decoded.

There are a number of channels that we use to communicate with others. These channels or methods tend to correspond to particular senses such as sight and hearing and, for each channel that we use, there is a method or way that facilitates its use best. We all communicate in many different forms, and the methods available for us to communicate are always increasing as information and communication technology develops, providing us with the opportunity to use multiple channels of communication to get our messages across. All the channels or methods have different advantages and disadvantages. When choosing a way to communicate, some of the aspects that you need to take into consideration are

- how much time is available;
- how many people you are communicating with;
- whether you want people to reply to you;
- whether you want people to be able to ask you questions;
- how much information you want to get from them;
- how much information you want to give them;
- how many senses (seeing, hearing, smelling) you need them to use for them to understand the information.

The way we choose to communicate with people depends on the channels of communication open to us. In a normal situation you do not notice yourself deciding on the considerations above when you communicate with someone. However, as someone working in a helping capacity in the health and social care fields, you do need to think more carefully about the best ways to communicate with someone else. You need to take into account their needs and not just yours and balance those needs against the needs of the organisation you work within. The message here is that once you start to unpick a communication and begin analysing the process you can start to appreciate the depth of meaning that lies behind the words and actions that you engage in. Even if you try not to interact with others you are still communicating with them. By hiding in the sluice or in the back room/office or just by simply staring out of the window you are communicating that you do not wish to interact with them. We communicate with all of our senses, our sight, hearing, smell and touch – in fact, we cannot not communicate.

Chapter 3

Introducing Transactional Analysis

Elaine Donnelly

Key themes

This chapter introduces Transactional Analysis and explores:

- what Transactional Analysis is;
- the concept of ego states;
- the Parent ego state;
- the Adult ego state;
- the Child ego state;
- transactions and analysing communication;
- life scripts;
- I'm OK, You're OK.

WHAT IS TRANSACTIONAL ANALYSIS?

Transactional Analysis (TA) is a way of describing in a simple format that is easily understood what takes place within people and between people. It is a way of studying and making sense of intra-personal and interpersonal relationships. It has at its core the belief that face-to-face communication is at the centre of human relationships, and if you are studying to develop your role in helping others it makes sense to include an overview of this theory in this book. What is offered here is my personal account of the work of Eric Berne, who was the originator of Transactional Analysis, and the work of other TA practitioners.

Eric Berne (1910–70) trained as a psychoanalyst and developed many theories during his lifetime. His work included six books (listed in the References) and he wrote many articles and edited the journal *Transactional Analysis Bulletin* until his death. He was the original founder of the International Transactional Analysis Association (TAA), which is the recognised professional body for therapists who use TA techniques in their psychotherapeutic work. TA is very popular in the United States and was popular here in the United Kingdom during the 1960s and '70s. It is pleasing to see that it is again becoming popular, not only as a therapeutic technique but as a method for improving communications in organisations. You can study short courses on TA all over the country and some universities offer Masters-level degrees and doctorate programmes of study. For me the work of Eric Berne removed the mystery that surrounds psychotherapy. Semenoff (cited in Klein, 1980) comments that 'what Berne proposed was essentially Freud without the unconscious'. TA uses everyday language resulting in an understandable theory that can be used by anyone as a method for understanding human communication and relationships.

THE CONCEPT OF EGO STATES

At the heart of TA is the notion that our personality is made up of three alter ego states. Berne (1961) called these ego states Parent, Adult and Child (PAC). These terms have specific definitions within this theory and care should be taken to avoid misinterpretation with the everyday terms of parent, adult and child. Each ego state is said to have different qualities and different patterns of behaviour and, to be a fully functioning person, we need to have access to all of our ego states.

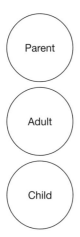

The Parent ego state is said to develop in us as children via the messages (teaching) we receive. It contains a great deal of recorded material that plays back and directs our behaviour. It is everything that we were taught.

The Adult ego state can be described as the thinking part of the self. It stores facts and processes information generated from within ourselves and from the external environment. It is everything that is thought.

The Child ego state holds all of the feelings that we have experienced in our lives. From anxiety to anger, depression to despair, happiness and joy. It holds all our fun and laughter. It is everything that is felt.

This simple model of a personality can provide us with an incredibly powerful tool to analyse our own and others' behaviour. You can spot which ego state someone is operating from simply by the words that they use, their tone of voice and their gestures and behaviour. Analysing ego states is referred to as Structural Analysis and analysing transactions, i.e. those interactions that take place between people, is referred to as Transactional

Analysis which we shall explore later. Let's move on and give you an opportunity to see if you can spot ego state characteristics and determine which is which. The details that follow are by no means comprehensive but they do give you an idea of how to spot which ego state you are accessing either in your own head or observing in others.

The Parent ego state

The Parent ego state is full of moral messages stored as recordings and it has set patterns of behaving. Just like a parent it can be loving and doting and succour us throughout our lives. The Parent ego state can nurture and protect the self and others that it communicates with and has relationships with, but it can also spoil us by being over-indulgent. It can be controlling and help maintain order but it can also be condemning, critical and harsh. The Parent ego state within us reflects the qualities of those people who cared for us as small children. It will include parents and other people who acted as care givers such as grandparents, aunts and uncles, teachers, ministers of religion and people you admired and adored.

Reflection

Take some time to consider some of the people who were important to you in your life when you were a small child.

- Can you recall any of the things that they regularly said?
- What were the underlying messages behind the things that they said?
- Do you live by those messages now?

I am happy to share one of my messages with you. My mother always used to say 'no matter how hard it is, you've just got to get on with it'. I live by that message now. There have been times in my life when things have been incredibly difficult but, guess what, no matter how difficult it has been I just 'dust myself down' (another one of her sayings) and get on with it. My mother was, in the main, a very controlling parent; perhaps she needed to be with six children. I believe her mother was very controlling too, but I always knew I was loved and that she would sort things out for me if I got into difficulty. Please don't think that I had a perfect childhood as I didn't and I don't believe that a perfect childhood exists. In contrast to that supportive controlling way that she had there were times when she was incredibly critical and patronising, but using TA as a framework to analyse her behaviour and my responses to it have enabled me to understand what took place between us and that insight into my own behaviour has enabled me to make alternative choices in the parenting of my own children.

What about you? It is likely that the things you value now are very similar to the things those people who were around you when you were small held dear. How often do you find yourself behaving in ways or saying the things that people did or said to you when you were small? I sometimes open my mouth and my mother's words spill out. My reaction is 'goodness, who invited mother into the conversation?' Now that I have that insight into my own behaviour I can choose to be like her or not as the case may be. With that insight I now have the opportunity to change. Personal reflection on your own internal dialogues and examining where they came from and what they mean to you can enable you to develop your communication and relationship skills with others.

Writing activity

Using the simple framework provided here, detail what you would identify as the characteristics of the Parent ego state.

Characteristics	Nurturing/Spoiling Parent	Controlling/Critical Parent
Words used		
Tone of voice		
Behaviours		
Attitude		

Parent ego state words

The Parent ego state uses words like: 'you must', 'you mustn't', 'you should', 'you shouldn't', 'you ought', 'you ought not', 'that's good', 'good boy', 'good girl', 'bad boy', 'bad girl', 'that's bad', 'just get on', 'just leave it', 'that's right', 'that's wrong', 'don't do this', 'don't do that', 'do this', 'do that', 'never mind', 'hurry up', 'stop that', 'mummy will do that', 'well done darling' and so on.

Tone of voice

The Parent ego state uses two main tones, that of concern and that of authority. The voice can be either soft or loud, patronising or helpful.

Have you heard irate parents in the supermarket speak to their children through clenched teeth? They are so incensed and angry but they are saving the admonishment until the child is at home and away from the public eye. The tone can often suggest a different communication from the words used.

Behaviours

The Parent ego state is also identifiable by its behaviours. Gestures, smiles, frowns, folded arms, open arms, pointing fingers, raised eyebrow, etc. are all markers of a Parent ego state.

Attitude

The attitude displayed by a Parent ego state is what makes the whole communication tie together, or not, as the case may be. It can be giving and caring or moralistic, patronising and judgemental. It can be authoritarian and controlling or facilitating and helpful. The ego state's attitude is reflected in the words, tone, behaviour and other subtle paralanguage used within the communication and the relationship.

The Adult ego state

Writing activity

Use the same process as before and identify the characteristics of the Adult ego state.

Characteristics	Adult ego state
Words used	
Tone of voice	
Behaviours	
Attitude	

The Adult is that part of you that has gathered knowledge, experience and skills throughout your life. In the small child the Adult ego state is in a state of development and is sometimes called the Little Professor in that it acts on instinct, without the full experience and knowledge that you have as an adult, and often that instinct pays off. How we learn is the subject of psychological theory and I find Piaget's (1977) schematic process of development useful in explaining how we learn to know and understand the world by building on past experiences, and the way in which we think qualitatively differently as a child compared with when we are an adult.

The Adult ego state learns how things work. It is the thinking part of the self. I think the perfect Adult ego state is presented by the character Mr Spock from the television and film series *Star Trek*. The character often considers his human colleagues as 'highly illogical' when they use emotional intelligence to help them get to the root of an intergalactic problem or when they express emotion such as love and hate. Please remember that Mr Spock is from another planet and as such does not represent a fully functioning human being, but I do call him to mind when I am struggling with an issue that needs level-headedness and rational, logical thought.

The Adult ego state is the bit of you that gets you organised. It makes plans, it formulates decisions and it weighs things up and remembers things. The Adult ego state relies on the direction of the parent and all those 'tape recorded' messages about what is right and what is wrong and it takes into account the feelings of the child. It has an executive function in deciding what to do.

Recognising the Adult ego state

Like the Parent ego state, the Adult ego state is recognisable by the words, the tone, the behaviour and attitude used within an interaction. It asks questions like 'how?', 'when?', 'where?', 'who?' and 'why?'. It uses phases such as 'that is interesting; mmmmm I think that's a possibility, maybe we could try that out'. The Adult ego state is calm, reflective and thoughtful and its attitude is one of being prepared to examine the facts, of level-headedness and rationality. The behaviour of the Adult ego state includes thoughtful looks, thinking behaviour, rubbing the face, scratching the head, gesturing possibilities with hand movements, itemising things and writing things down.

The Adult ego state can influence our Parent ego state by evaluating new information and instigating change through that reflective process. It can help to keep the emotions of the Child ego state in check but it is important to remember that the Adult ego state is a reflection of everything that has happened to us, so change is not always as easy as it sounds.

You will be familiar with sayings such as 'mind over matter' and you may believe that, if thought determines our behaviour, changing how people think will change their behaviour. However, if you have ever tried to change people's behaviour by using factual information and thoughts alone, you are likely to have been only partially successful. Let's examine that a little further.

Reflection

How would you set about helping someone to give up smoking? You might also consider looking at other examples of risk-taking behaviour.

Changing someone's perception and behaviour isn't as easy as it sounds. You could try to give them new information so their Adult ego state could process the same, but it is more than likely that you will hit all sorts of obstacles that arise from the person's willingness to think things through.

Everyone knows that smoking poses an enormous health risk to the individual and those around them. To me the facts are quite clear, so why don't people stop smoking? Child ego state, feelings, ingrained patterns of behaviour and attitudes all need to be addressed. Just as you can rationalise the ways in which smoking is bad for them, they may rationalise that smoking didn't kill 'old Mr Smith' from down the road, who smoked 40 a day and lived till he was a 103 years old, so it's not going to kill them and, besides which, they like it. The key to change is that people need to commit themselves to change and will need much more than factual information. We'll come back to this later.

The Child ego state

Please don't assume that the word 'Child' means child-like. To be a fully functioning person we all need to be able to access our Child ego state. When we are born our Child ego state is all that we have. It is through the process of the 'parenting' of others that we develop other ego states. Berne (1961) argued that the Child ego state, in many ways, is the best bit of us. It is creative and joyful, it has fun and can be spontaneous, it is loving and uninhibited, it is curious, and in awe of the world. Not to have any of these aspects to our personality would leave the world bereft of all the things that have come out of these positive qualities. However, just as the Child has the potential for all these things, it is subject to its 'parenting' (I use the word 'parenting' loosely here, as I mean the people who are responsible for parenting or care-giving but they may not be the child's parents in the biological sense).

The people who 'parent' the small child are all-powerful to that child and if their parenting skills, which are located and recorded in their Parent ego state, are not appropriate or fall short in some way, as a consequence of external or even internal events, the child still has to survive. To do so, the child adapts his/her behaviour. Adapted behaviour can be seen in all of us. Children figure out how to get what it is that they want, and their behaviour may please or displease their parents but they are able to work out how to get what they want. If the child wants attention it works out the easiest and quickest way to get it. That way may involve kicking and screaming or doing something naughty like biting their baby sister, or it may be smiling nicely and looking up through ultra-long lashes and being adorable. Either way attention is the result. That attention may not be delivered as we would like it to be, it may involve negative and harmful consequences, but attention is attention to the needy child. Our Child ego state adapts and learns how to manipulate situations, learns how to smile when unhappy, learns how to be cute, how to charm people and how to maintain the status quo. Not to adapt could result in tragedy for the personality as a whole, if not for the person, as it needs to be recognised that adaptive behaviour, while necessary to survive, can be very destructive and can result in devastating consequences.

The Child ego state holds all the feelings of childhood and carries them into adulthood where they continue to affect how we feel about ourselves and how we relate to others.

Writing activity

Repeat the same process as before and see if you can identify the Child ego state characteristics.

Characteristics	Natural/Free Child	Adapted Child
Words used		
Tone of voice		
Behaviours		
Attitude		

Child ego state words

The Child ego state often uses baby talk to express itself. It uses words like: 'help me', 'I can't do this on my own', 'this is my best day', 'my worst day', 'I can', 'I can't', 'I won't', 'I want', 'no', 'please', 'thank you', 'yippee', 'hooray', 'brilliant', 'yes', 'now', 'never'. Fitting them into what is free and what is adapted is a little tricky, but tone of voice is usually the give away. Tone of voice can often be in the extreme: screaming, shouting, excited, joyful, high-pitched or quiet, whining and pathetic.

Child ego state behaviours

Child ego state behaviours reflect the emotions and feelings being experienced at the time. Folded arms, looking sad, giggling, not being able to give or maintain eye contact and hiding the face. Temper tantrums which involve thrashing arms and legs on the floor, etc. are common expressions of a Child ego state. Learning how to control extreme emotions is difficult but most of us manage it, although I do know a few adults who would love to kick and scream every now and then. The Child ego state knows how to hit your 'buttons' as they are able, through their Little Professor, to suss you out and how to get you to react.

Child ego state attitudes

Attitudes differ according to whether we are operating from our Free or Natural Child or from our Adapted Child. Child ego states can be free of inhibition, spirited, happy-go-lucky, volatile, manipulative, sly, cunning, compliant or defiant, all rolled up into one.

According to TA, 'good parenting' is the key to healthy Child ego states (Whitton, 1993) but healthy does not mean free or natural all of the time. We have to learn to self regulate our behaviour and take our cues from others in order to fit in with our social group. Sometimes 'good parenting' is not possible because of our own parents' Parent ego state. It may be damaged or incomplete. It is, after all, a product of its own experiences and maybe they did not have their emotional needs met when they were small. Being in our Parent ego state is comfortable as all those pre-recorded messages need little thinking about and little effort to sustain, but we can change those recorded ways of being through reflection and analysis of self and the relationships we have with others.

That was quite a tricky concept to explain and I did labour some of the points but it is important when using this framework to understand yourself and others, and not to attribute blame, as it takes two people to make a relationship. That brings me on nicely to transactions and communications between people.

TRANSACTIONS BETWEEN PEOPLE

Alongside Structural Analysis of the personality, Eric Berne (1961) identified the process for analysing conversations between two or more people
as the 'analysis of the transactional framework'. A transaction is said to be
the means by which we receive and transmit 'strokes'. A stroke is defined
as a 'unit of recognition' and strokes are essential to functional living. The
achievement of strokes motivates our behaviour. According to this theory
we all seek recognition from others. Recognition from others validates who
we are. Transmitting a stroke to another person can be something as simple
as saying 'good morning', and our reward is that they will say 'good morning' back, so validating that we are worthy of being recognised and
responded to. When we give strokes we expect to be paid back.

Complementary transactions

A transaction is transmitted and received via an ego state, and transactions
are said to be either complementary, crossed or have at their core an ulterior motive. I've used one diagram (Figure 4) to show three examples of
complementary transactions between the different ego states.

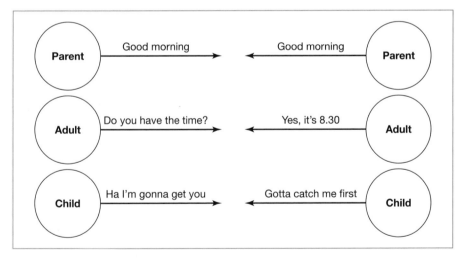

Figure 4 Complementary transactions between the different ego states

The Parent to Parent ego states are passing the time of day, sharing normal
polite conversation. The Adult ego state is seeking information from
another and receives the same. The Child issues an invitation to play
which is accepted.

We are expected to pay back strokes by interacting with the person who
gave us the stroke initially. A stroke may be a nod of the head or a series of

strokes during a long discussion about global warming, but communication needs to be responded to in order for it to continue. If it is not responded to, the person who initiated the interaction often feels aggrieved. For example, if I say 'good morning' to a colleague and they don't respond I feel a bit put out. The Child ego state in my head says 'I must have done something' or 'she doesn't really like me' and I am left feeling embarrassed and sad. Later, I find myself sitting at the same table and I say, 'I said "hello" this morning and you totally ignored me. Have I offended you?' She responds immediately, 'Oh gosh no. I am so sorry, my head was elsewhere this morning. I forgot my diary. I didn't see you. Anyway, how are you doing? You look absolutely great.' Not only do I get an apology and an explanation, but I also get an extra stroke in the form of a compliment. The communication between us can continue as she has paid back the stroke.

What if I hadn't caught up with her at lunch time but met someone else who had also been ignored by that person that morning? You can imagine the conversation. We talk about her ignoring us and decide she must be troubled by something and we agree to make a deliberate attempt to go find her and offer her our support, or we condemn her for being rude and ignorant and decide to ignore her in future. (Sounds like a Child ego state in play here.) If a transaction is complementary it can continue. Figure 5 gives other examples:

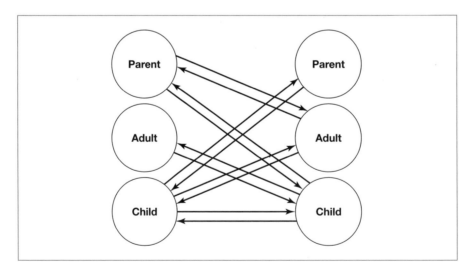

Figure 5 Examples of complementary transactions (you can make up the dialogue for each)

Crossed transactions

To be a complementary transaction one ego state must communicate with another and the response must come from the ego state the transaction was aimed at. This can go very wrong and, when it does, it is called a crossed transaction. See the following examples in Figure 6.

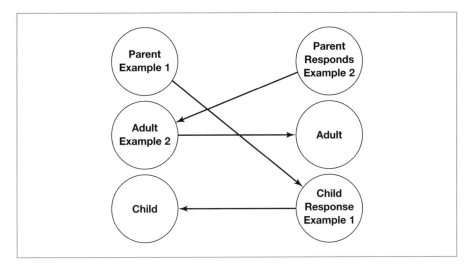

Figure 6 Crossed transactions

In the examples above we can see a Parent ego state (Example 1) communicating with another person's Child ego state, shown via the diagrammatic line. It may be useful to note that the Parent ego state is likely to be a parent and the Child ego state is likely to be an actual child in this transaction. The Child ego state, rather than responding in a complementary way at the same level, chooses to respond by aiming its transaction to the other person's Child ego state in an adapted manner (Response 1).

Adding the following dialogue to the diagrammatic lines may help you to make sense of this crossed transaction.

Parent 1. When you have finished there you can come and have your tea.
Child 1. I don't want your stinky tea. I hate you and I hate tea, leave me alone.

The second example is that of an Adult ego state seeking information from another Adult ego state, but surprisingly the other person's Parent ego state responds. I've provided some dialogue as before but you may wish to add your own.

Adult 2. Do you know where the digital timer is?
Parent 2. Why do you expect me to know where everything is? You had it last.

Again, the response was not what was expected.

Crossed transactions often result in leaving people upset and the communication that was initiated ends as the invitation to come for tea or the request for information about the digital timer is left aside.

Berne (1972) calculated there were mathematically 72 types of crossed interactions and nine types of complementary interactions. I haven't been able to work them all out but, given his expertise, I believe it is so.

Ulterior or covert transactions

The final type of transaction that Berne proposed is described as an ulterior or covert transaction. Here there is a social message in what is being said but there is a hidden message too (see Figure 7).

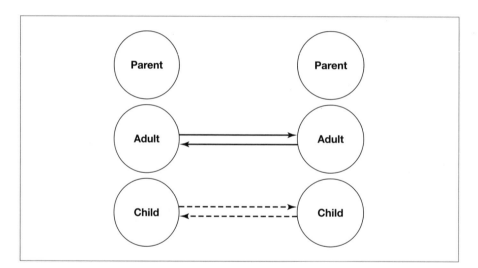

Figure 7 An ulterior or covert transaction

In this transaction the top line transaction represents the social level of the message sent. Adult to Adult: 'Come up to the gallery and see my etchings …'.The response on a social level is Adult to Adult: 'Oh yes, that would be lovely'.

You can see in this transaction that there is another level of communication – Child to Child – referred to by Berne (1972) as the 'psychological' or 'covert level'. This sort of transaction has a psychological hook. In this example, that hook had a sexual connotation that has been recognised and accepted by the responder. However, the initiator took a risk as the responder could have responded from Critical Parent to Child with a comment such as: 'I don't particularly like etchings as I find them immature and brash.' The transaction would then be a crossed one and the communication ended.

LIFE SCRIPTS

Another theory of TA is that of life scripts. It is suggested that we, as small children, write our own life script and then live according to its principles. A life script can be explored through the process of story telling. Whitton (1993) provides an exercise to help explore life scripts. The following exercise is adapted from his text, *What is Transactional Analysis? A Personal and Practical Guide.*

Reflection and writing activity

1. Think about your life as a small child and try to piece together a short story that describes your experience of the world and who you are. What happened when you were born? What did your parents say? Who gave you your name? Where do you fit in the family?
2. Write down a story that reflects your life. 500 words will do.
3. Reflecting on that story:
   - are you the main character or do you have a cameo part?
   - are you the hero or a drudge?
   - is your story similar to other stories that you were fond of as a child?

The analysis of all this is up to you, but I hope it gives you an opportunity to think about who you are and how your childhood has influenced you as an adult. Perhaps it even helps to explain why you have chosen to be in the helping profession.

According to Whitton (1993), writing your life script took place before you were five years old. Life scripts influence how we receive and transmit messages to ourselves and to others. Our life script determines our decisions about what messages to accept and what to ignore. Life scripts, according to Whitton, are 'essential for the child to survive'. We do hear stories of children who have been seriously abused and neglected but somehow they have raised themselves above all that negativity and become successful adults. According to this theory, these children wrote fantasy life scripts in their heads and used them to protect themselves from what went on around them. In this way they could refuse to receive negative messages and refuse to allow them to damage their personality, even though they may have been damaged physically. Positive messages would have been swept up, stored and cherished.

I'm OK, You're OK

Very early in the writing of our life scripts we are said to make a decision about whether or not we are OK. The saying 'I'm OK, You're OK' may be familiar to you, and it originates from the title of a book written by Thomas Harris in 1969. Harris was an eminent psychiatrist and psychoanalyst and, as a TA practitioner, his work detailed how we respond to ourselves and to the world. Harris constructed the 'OK Corral' (see Figure 8) as a way of explaining people's Life Positions and concluded that, once we have made our life position decision, all our transactions are made in such a way as to maintain the same position.

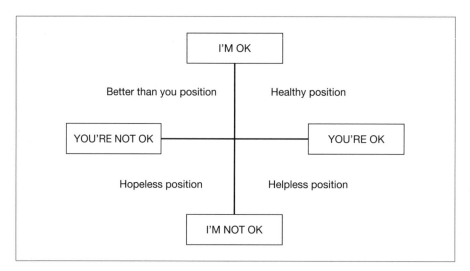

Figure 8 The OK Corral (Harris, 1969 and 1985)

Where do you sit within the OK Corral? Each of us has a preferred way of being, and our transactions with the self and with others project this way of being. See if you can work out the following:

1. Which position do the words 'Do as I say' come from?
2. Which position do the words 'It's not fair' come from?
3. Which position do the words 'That was fun, let's do it again' come from?
4. Which position do the words 'Nobody can help me' come from?

I have no doubt you were able to work those positions out accurately as each ego state is clearly recognisable within the OK Corral, but I've included the answers at the end of the chapter for you to check.

That we make decisions about our life script and our life position at such an early stage is quite remarkable. According to TA theory we do review those decisions during adolescence but most of us stay the same and live our lives according to our script, taking selected strokes and messages as a reinforcement of our life position. On an intra-personal level we call on those messages to help maintain the *status quo* even though they are not always healthy messages.

We are not always accurate in our understanding of life and we don't like change. Change brings with it anxiety and uncertainty and many people stay where they are, despite terrible consequences, as it is what they know. The Adult ego state within us is often contaminated by the other two ego states and rationalises situations in a flawed way, so maintaining life as it knows it to be.

Analysing transactions, life scripts and positions is fascinating and Eric Berne's explanation of the personality is easily understood. Once you learn how to identify which ego state you are operating from, you can understand why you behave and feel as you do. You could even choose to change your transaction by switching to another ego state. For example, you could move out of Critical Parent and stop criticising the children and join in their fun via your Child ego state. Knowing what ego state another person is in can help you to respond more effectively. You may even be able to intervene in such a way as to help the person understand which ego state they are operating from.

This chapter has introduced you to some of the principles of Transactional Analysis. TA provides a common language that you can share with others including family, friends, work colleagues and people that you seek to help. It is an effective communication tool as well as a psychotherapeutic technique and there are lots of texts available to read and courses to attend.

Reading activity

You need to read other people's accounts of Transactional Analysis and TA practitioners are generally incredibly generous in sharing their material. All of the books in the References are still in print and there are several online sites that are worth having a look at such as, for example **www.itaa-net.org** and **www.ta-tutor.com**

Answers to Life Position questions

1. Which position do the words 'Do as I say' come from?
   Critical Parent in an I'm OK, You're not OK position.
2. Which position do the words 'It's not fair' come from?
   Adapted Child in a You're OK, I'm not OK position.
3. Which position do the words 'That was fun, let's do it again' come from?

Free Child in an I'm OK, You're OK position.

4. Which position do the words 'Nobody can help me' come from?

Adapted Child in an I'm not OK, You're not OK position.

Chapter 4

An Introduction to Counselling Skills

Lindsey Neville

Key themes

This chapter explores

- the difference between counselling and counselling skills;

- theoretical frameworks of counselling;

- learning counselling skills;

- core conditions and the work of Carl Rogers;

- the six-stage category intervention model of John Heron;

- the three-stage model of Gerard Egan;

- the skills of active listening, attending, reflecting, paraphrasing and summarising;

- ethical and boundary issues;

- the perspective of those who use our services.

In this chapter you will begin to explore the use of counselling skills within the 'helping' professions. It is important to understand first a little of what counselling is, how it differs from the use of counselling skills and how both counselling and the use of counselling skills may help service users. Reid (2004) explores the work of counsellors in a variety of health and social care, education, voluntary and independent settings.

THE DIFFERENCE BETWEEN COUNSELLING AND COUNSELLING SKILLS

Counselling is sometimes called a talking therapy. It is a helping activity in which the counsellor listens to the client and helps them to tell their story or difficulty. It takes place when a counsellor and client agree to spend time together, the purpose being to help the client to talk about something that troubles them. The purpose of counselling is to help and support the person to move emotionally from one place to another. Counselling is not about giving advice or telling people what to do. The British Association for Counselling and Psychotherapy [BACP] defines counselling as:

> A contractual arrangement when a counsellor meets a client in privacy and confidence to explore a difficulty, distress they may be experiencing, perhaps their dissatisfaction with life or loss of a sense of direction or purpose.
>
> (BACP, 2006)

Counselling usually takes place in a structured setting. The client and counsellor meet together in private, usually for an hour at the same time each week. It is important to draw a distinction between counselling and friendship. Friendship is usually a two-way process in which both parties might benefit from a sharing of thoughts and feelings. Counsellors rarely share their own thoughts and feelings but work with those of others. Geldard and Geldard (2003) explore the differences in more depth and their text *Counselling Skills in Everyday Life* offers a straightforward approach to understanding some of the key issues. Counselling sessions are confidential, with very few important exceptions that will be explained later in this chapter. In the past, counselling was always a face-to-face activity but, in recent years, telephone and e.mail counselling have become more popular.

Reflection

- Can you think why telephone and e.mail counselling may have become more popular?
- Can you identify any of the counselling services available via these channels?

It is not the aim of this book to explore counselling and its many formats in depth, but to facilitate an understanding of the difference between counselling and using counselling skills. Many of my students who would like to understand more about the nature of counselling have found it helpful to read *Counselling for Toads* by De Board (1998). It is an easy and very enjoyable text that manages to explain a great deal about the theory of counselling by using the story of *The Wind in the Willows* (Grahame, 1908).

How helpful counselling has been can be difficult to determine. In the past, research in this area has been limited but, more recently, the subject has become the focus of a number of studies. The Department of Health (2001) found that counselling may benefit service users who are adjusting to life events, illnesses, disabilities and losses. The McLeod review *Counselling in the Workplace* (2001) found that counselling intervention had a 'positive impact on job commitment, work function, job satisfaction and substance misuse' (p. 8) and noted that levels of sickness and absence fell by 25 to 50 per cent in some areas. Lambert (2003) found a considerable amount of evidence that showed that psychological therapies were generally effective and the National Audit Office (2006) found that Employee Assistance Programmes were effective in reducing sickness levels.

Theoretical frameworks of counselling

Although there are a lot of shared beliefs about counselling, there are different theoretical frameworks. This means that, over time, different practitioners will have constructed different ways of making sense of their work with clients. So a conceptual framework is a way of thinking or theorising about the work. You might also see these referred to as theoretical frameworks or perspectives. It helps to understand a little about them because these theoretical approaches are at the very core of the helping profession's relationship with service users.

Trevethick (2000) uses the words of Susser (1968) to highlight the importance of theory to practice:

> to practise without theory is to sail an uncharted sea; theory without practice is not to set sail at all (p. 14).

The theoretical frameworks that we have chosen as most applicable to the application of counselling skills include:

- the Psychodynamic approach;
- the Behavioural approach;
- the Cognitive approach;
- the Person-centred approach;
- the Humanistic approach;
- Neuro-Linguistic Programming (NLP).

Practitioners who use a mix of different frameworks are said to have an eclectic approach. Exploring these in detail is not part of this text but the Further Reading section contains some texts that will help you read more about the conceptual frameworks of counselling if you would like to further your study.

Research has shown that some of these approaches are more useful than others for working with specific conditions. Counsellors use a variety of advanced counselling skills, within one of these conceptual frameworks, to help clients explore their difficulties and perhaps reach some kind of better understanding for themselves. These skills are not unique to professional therapists but are common to most helping relationships in both voluntary and statutory sectors and we will discuss them at more length later in this chapter. Regardless of the counselling approach, most counsellors would agree that it is the relationship between counsellor and client that is the most important aspect of counselling.

In the past some organisations such as universities, colleges and schools have tried to make counselling part of their disciplinary procedures. For example, those with challenging behaviour might have been sent to see the counsellor. In more recent years we have come to understand that there are no benefits in sending someone for counselling. The person must want to engage in the process and form a partnership with the counsellor or therapist. There are many ways in which an individual can see a counsellor.

- By asking your GP, as some surgeries will have their own counsellor.
- Through a voluntary organisation. These are usually established to meet the needs of clients with a specific concern, for example, RELATE, which supports those with relationship issues. There are also organisations that support those who have experienced sexual abuse, domestic violence, or drug, gambling or alcohol addiction.
- Many employers offer counselling schemes for their employees.
- Most schools, colleges and universities have a resident counsellor.
- Some counsellors work independently of any organisation and advertise themselves privately, perhaps through their accrediting organisation such as, for example, BACP (British Association for Counselling and Psychotherapy), or through the internet or listings in telephone directories.

Sometimes these services are free to the client (perhaps those offered by employers or a primary care trust, or some voluntary organisations). Where counselling services are offered by private counsellors a fee is paid by the client for each session. Some counsellors have sliding scales of payment for those on low incomes. Some voluntary organisations that offer counselling will ask for a donation. Voluntary counselling organisations such as RELATE are also training organisations and, therefore, the counsellors may be at different stages of training.

Many large organisations employ their own counsellor. Other employers might pay for the services of an Employee Assistance Programme (EAP). EAP providers offer experienced counsellors who respond to the needs of a workforce. The service is usually confidential and they aim to offer their clients access to experienced counsellors over the phone, 24 hours a day, seven days a week, with face-to-face counselling where appropriate.

It is important to note that at the time of writing (June 2007) counsellors are not required to be professionally registered, unlike many other health and social care practitioners such as nurses, doctors and social workers. However, the government is currently planning to introduce statutory regulation for all psychological therapists, which includes counsellors, applied psychologists and psychotherapists (Department of Health (DoH), 2007). This means that, at the moment, anyone can call themselves a counsellor with any level of training or none. There are, however, a number of professional bodies for those who work in this area. Those accredited by a professional organisation will have to adhere to its minimum standards in training, experience, supervision and professional development.

Reading activity

In your helping position you may find yourself being asked for further advice and details on how best to get counselling. The following web references are worth a visit and will provide you with more information. The British Association for Counselling and Psychotherapy (BACP) is available at **www.bacp.co.uk** Counselling and Psychotherapy in Scotland (COSCA) is available via **www.cosca.org.uk** The United Kingdom Register of Counsellors (UKRC) is a list of those counsellors who have achieved recognition by an accrediting organisation. This can be found at **www.ukrconline.org.uk**

There is a wide range of qualifications and experience among counsellors. Some counselling organisations are also training organisations and, as such, counsellors will be at different stages of training. Anyone who is practising as a counsellor should ideally have at least a Diploma in Counselling and some counsellors may have a graduate or postgraduate qualification in counselling.

The duration of counselling will depend upon the nature of the difficulty and the approach used by the counsellor. It would be usual for the counsellor to discuss their expectations with the client at the first session though, of course, the time frame can change from individual to individual and as understanding deepens or issues develop. Counselling does not go on for years and is more likely to last between 4 and 12 sessions.

Counsellors are all supervised. Supervision is the process by which counsellors reflect on their cases with, usually, a counsellor who is more experienced than they are and who may have had additional training as a supervisor. Ideally, supervision should take place once a month and last for one and a half hours. It gives the counsellor a chance to explore issues connected with each case, to have the input of another counsellor and to have an opportunity to discuss the impact of the work on their own wellbeing. The supervisor shares a responsibility for ensuring that the counsellor is fit to practise. The supervisor is bound by the same confidentiality agreement as the counsellor.

Reflection

Sally is a service user who thinks that she needs counselling. What issues does she need to consider when choosing a counsellor? It might be helpful to discuss this with a colleague and compare your thoughts.

Sally will find it beneficial to ask a range of questions before making a decision about which counsellor to see. A wealth of information can be obtained through any of the websites given in this chapter and these will help inform the decision-making progress. She might ask:

- Which theoretical framework is most appropriate for the issue I wish to address?
- What qualifications and experience does the counsellor have?
- How much will it cost?
- Does the counsellor have regular supervision?
- Is the counsellor a member of a professional body such as the BACP?

All of these are important considerations before choosing a counsellor.

Learning counselling skills

Counselling skills are the tools of the professional counsellor but these skills can also be learned and used by anyone who is in a helping relationship. They are used to help someone to tell us their story. We can use the skills in our relationships with friends and family or in our working relationships with colleagues and service users. Many of the readers of this book will already have and use a number of the skills within their personal and professional lives.

We all see the world differently and the underlying aim of using counselling skills is to try to see the world as others see it. For those who work in health and social care settings these skills will form the foundation for all of your professional interactions and enable you to build a reputation as an effective communicator.

Look at the W.E. Hill cartoon below. Describe what you see. When I show this to a group of students they may perceive it differently. The reason for this is that both images are present in the picture. The cartoon is called *My Wife and my Mother-in-law*. Do you see an old lady or a young lady? For many people the images will alternate but it can be difficult to see the second image once you have focused on the first. Try putting the picture a little further away from you.

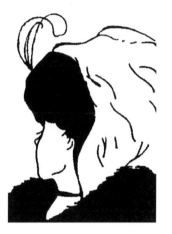

It may help you to see both if you know that the mouth of the old lady is the choker necklace of the young lady, and the chin of the young lady is the nose of the old woman. In this exercise we see the image differently even though we are all looking at the same thing. The same can be true of how we see experiences and feelings. There are other examples of this kind of image, e.g. Rubin's Vase.

There are a number of theorists whose work impacts upon the use of counselling skills but, for the purposes of this text, I have identified three key theorists whose work is helpful in informing the use of counselling skills in health and social care settings.

Core conditions of counselling and the work of Carl Rogers

Rogers' theory has at its centre the belief that each individual has the capability and the intent to make the most of their own life. He calls this an 'actualising tendency'. Rogers (2002) believes that, in order to enable individuals to move towards this actualisation (being the person we really are), helping relationships need to have three core conditions:

1. empathy;
2. congruence;
3. unconditional positive regard.

Where these conditions are evident in the relationship between service user and helper, an effective partnership will be established and the client will feel that they are empowered and understood, and that they can trust the person they are talking to.

Empathy

Empathy is often confused with sympathy, but it is very different. Sympathy is showing that you care and understand about people's problems. Empathy is the ability to imagine what it must be like to be in someone's personal situation (*Cambridge Learners Dictionary*, 2007). An empathic person thinks about what it would be like to see the world as the other person sees it.

Congruence

If we are congruent with another person it means that we are real with them, that we are showing them our true self. To do this we need to be comfortable with who we are and not pretend to be someone we are not.

Unconditional positive regard

Having unconditional positive regard for another person means that we accept them as they are and that we do not judge their behaviour, attitudes, values or beliefs. This requires that we set aside our own attitudes, values and beliefs so that they do not colour our relationship with service users.

Often these skills are associated with older practitioners, as they come with knowledge of self and life experience. For this reason many organisations have been reluctant to take on younger applicants for counselling training courses. This is not necessarily a position that I would support as, in my teaching on counselling skills courses, I have been privileged to meet students of all ages who have the ability to demonstrate these 'core conditions'. Later in this chapter you will learn more about how these three 'core conditions' can be achieved in our work with people who use your services.

The six-stage category intervention model of John Heron

John Heron established his framework for counselling interventions in the mid-1970s. His work was inspired by that of Blake and Mouton in the early 1970s. Heron's model focuses mainly on one-to-one interventions between helper and service user. An intervention, within this context, is the process of getting involved, of taking part in a process. If a helper makes an intervention, they will be offering something to a discussion. The intervention can be verbal or non-verbal. For example, a service user who is telling you a difficult story will find it encouraging if you intervene occasionally by showing listening behaviours such as nodding.

Heron (2003) categorises six interventions that he feels are appropriate in counselling. The model helps us to identify our own helping style. Certain styles will also be more appropriate in some settings than others. He suggests that there are six kinds of helping behaviour and divides these into two groups, 'authoritative' and 'facilitative' interventions.

Authoritative interventions

In this group of interventions the helper is taking some responsibility for the service user. Interventions are clearly identifiable in that they will be:

1. confronting – this is used to raise awareness of a behaviour or attitude which may be limiting the service user;
2. prescriptive – this directs actions;
3. informative – this gives knowledge or information.

Facilitative interventions

This group of interventions is more about empowering the service user and involves using interventions that are:

4. catalytic – this promotes problem-solving and self-discovery;
5. supportive – this affirms worth and value;
6. cathartic – this enables the expression of strong emotion.

Reflection

Consider the following types of intervention that might be used in health and social care settings and then identify which of Heron's intervention categories would be appropriate.

1. Guidance from a health care professional about lowering blood cholesterol levels.
2. A staff appraisal interview with a colleague whose work has not been to the expected standard.
3. A counsellor working with a client who wants to change their behaviour.
   - Can you identify the sort of interventions you use in the course of your work?
   - Are those interventions effective or would they benefit from further consideration?
   - Think about an intervention you used today. Could you have used an alternative approach?
   - What were the benefits of the approach you used?

Heron argues that we all use these interventions when responding to others and that careful consideration and reflection upon how we use them can result in those interventions being much more effective with those people that we seek to help.

The three-stage model of Gerard Egan

This model can be applied to work within health and social care settings as it aims to:

> help people become better at helping themselves in their everyday lives (Egan, 1998, pp. 7–8).

It encourages the empowerment of service users and is therefore compatible with contemporary perspectives of health and social care. Egan (1998) suggests that the model is at its most effective if applied using Rogers' (2002) Core Conditions, which were discussed earlier in this chapter.

Egan's model identifies three stages in the skilled helping relationship:

1. exploration;
2. understanding;
3. action.

Exploration

This is the first stage of the model and it involves encouraging the service user to first tell their story. It acknowledges the importance of the person really hearing their story perhaps for the first time as they speak the words aloud. The emphasis is on creating time and space for this to happen. The helper uses the counselling skills that are described in this chapter to facilitate the telling of the story.

Understanding

In this second stage of the model the helper supports the service user in trying to understand what they would like to change or do differently. It offers an opportunity to reflect on what has happened and, if they wish, to explore ways in which they might live their lives differently. They might be supported to identify a range of potential goals or actions.

Action

In this stage the helper can support the service user as they try to make changes based on their earlier understanding and reflection. These changes are achieved through the setting of goals. The service user can also be helped to explore the things that might hinder or support their development. In an ongoing relationship there can also be opportunities to experiment with different ways of behaving or being.

THE SKILLS OF COUNSELLING

Active listening

'Active listening' is an all-encompassing term used to describe the skills necessary to be an effective listener. Establishing a helping relationship depends on being able to create an environment in which people feel comfortable enough to share personal information. The key elements of a positive relationship in terms of acknowledging feelings, the impact of body language and the importance of effective listening are explored in Chapter 2. This chapter will add to those skills to enable you to develop your helping relationships.

Acknowledging feelings

Respecting people's feelings is central to being able to communicate with them. It's easy to go through our busy lives without really thinking about how we feel at any given moment. Working with people means that we need to consider how service users might be feeling, but we also need to be aware of our own emotional responses. Technological advances have made much of our communications quicker and easier, but emoticons in emails, text messages and instant messages have the effect of limiting our range of emotional descriptions. Being aware of our own feelings and being able to describe them helps us to acknowledge and work with the feelings of others. To do this we need to ensure that we have an extensive feelings-vocabulary and good observation skills. It is also important to be comfortable with people expressing strong emotions and this will be explored in more depth in Chapter 5.

Giving attention (this is sometimes called 'attending')

By this I mean that you need to demonstrate to the other person that they have your full attention; that you are listening to them. Some of the ways of doing this with body language and acknowledgement of feelings will be discussed in Chapter 6 but probably the most important way to demonstrate your attention to another person is to first of all consider the circumstances that would enable you to share personal information with another person. Sometimes people can do things that have the effect of closing us down rather than enabling us to open up.

Reflection

Try to remember a time when you have needed to talk over a difficult, sensitive or personal issue with a health care professional – perhaps your GP. What behaviour on the part of the GP helped you to feel more comfortable about discussing your concerns? Did s/he do or say anything that you found off-putting or which made the task harder?

It is likely that you felt more comfortable if your GP was welcoming and gave the impression that they had time for you and were interested in what you had to say. It helps if you feel that you have the other person's sole attention, that they don't answer the telephone or respond to other interruptions. Even furniture can send a message about the availability of the helper. A table between the two of you can create an emotional as well as physical barrier. A computer screen can also impact on the relationship by creating a more impersonal environment. It's helpful to apply this understanding that you gain from personal experience to your interactions with others.

Body language

Body language plays a key part in the messages that we send to those whom we work for and with. For example, I don't imagine there are many people who would find it easy to discuss personal matters with someone who doesn't look at them.

Paired activity

Ask someone to help you with this activity. You are going to tell them about the last 24 hours in your life, giving them as many details as you can in five minutes. Ask the other person to do everything they can to ignore you while remaining sitting next to you. You will probably have found that it was very difficult to keep going with your story while the other person showed no signs of listening. This tells us how important it is to demonstrate to people that we are listening.

Reflecting

Reflecting in this sense is the skill of being able to repeat to a client or service user a word or phrase that they have used. This enables them to hear the actual words that they have used. It gives the helper the opportunity to select what appears to be a significant word from among those used by the client. This has the effect of encouraging the client to focus on the word and consider it in more depth. For example, the client might say 'I have been feeling very lonely recently', so the helper might reflect the word 'lonely'. This is likely to encourage the client to reflect on their use of the word, consider it further and perhaps go on to say more about the loneliness.

Reflecting demonstrates that you are paying close attention to everything that the client says. The danger in using this skill is that it can come across as 'parroting', merely repeating a word without any focus or meaning. The real skill lies in the ability to reflect the word in a meaningful way. This is done mainly through tone of voice and body language.

Reflection

Consider the following sentences and choose a word that you might reflect to the client.

- 'I am frightened to go out at night.'
- 'I have been in a lot of pain recently.'
- 'Since my husband died I have found it difficult to manage.'

In each sentence try to choose the word that seems the most significant, that is the one that is most likely to encourage the client to say more.

Paraphrasing

Paraphrasing is the skill of identifying the meaning in what someone says. It can also involve picking up on the feelings underneath the words. For example, someone might say 'I haven't been sleeping. In the middle of the night I lie awake and all sorts of worries begin to overwhelm me. Then I can't get back to sleep and I am so tired which means I'm not coping with things in the day.' The helper might respond: 'You feel anxious when you aren't getting enough sleep.'

Activity

Try paraphrasing the following sentences:

- 'When my marriage failed, I felt that nothing would ever go right again and that I had let my children and my parents down'.
- 'I'm a really heavy smoker. I have never really thought about stopping but now that we are having a baby I feel that I should try'.
- 'I only ever wanted to have my own family and be a parent but I just didn't realise how hard it would be. It's exhausting and I never get time to myself, which makes me very bad-tempered, so I am always shouting at the children'.

Summarising

For my contemporaries the skill of summarising formed a large part of the English curriculum under the guise of what was called précis exercises. Basically, long passages had to be read and the key points identified and presented. The same principle applies in a counselling skills context. If you have created an environment based on the core conditions, service users will hopefully find it easy to talk to you and you may be on the receiving end of a great deal of information. There are several reasons that you might want to summarise what is said:

• To make sure that you have heard/understood correctly.
• To identify/separate key areas.
• To enable the service user to hear the issues that they have raised.

Reflection

Read the following case study.

'Paul walked out on me a year ago. Our relationship had always been very passionate or very angry but I just thought that was the way things were for us. I always wanted to be with him but he worked long hours so inevitably I spent a lot of time alone. Then when we were together I wanted a lot from him. He said that I was clingy which made me angry and things sometimes got violent between us. Either one or both of us would start throwing things. In the end things came to a head and a neighbour called the police. We were both so embarrassed. I thought that it would help us both change things for the better but he felt that it was the end rather than the new beginning that I had hoped for. It was his flat so I had to move out and find myself somewhere else to live. I have ended up sharing with some people that I don't really like. It's all made me feel so low. I've been to the doctor but all he did was give me a prescription for anti-depressants. All I want is to get Paul back but he doesn't answer my phone calls, texts or e.mails. I feel so lost and alone.'

1. What do you think are the key points in this story?
2. How might you summarise it to the service user?

It is important to identify the key elements of what has been said. In this case they appear to be:

- an intense, violent relationship has ended;
- now living with people she doesn't like;
- low mood.

So, you might summarise what the client has said as: 'Since your intense but sometimes violent relationship broke down a year ago you have had to move in with people that you don't like. Paul doesn't respond to your attempts to contact him and you are left feeling very low.'

Coping with silence

There is nothing wrong with having periods of silence when you are spending time with another person. They often occur naturally within conversations. People sometimes need time and space to consider what they want to say. If you feel that the length of silence has started to become uncomfortable for the service user you might like to reflect that by saying something like 'I wonder if it is difficult for you to know where to start'.

THE PERSPECTIVES OF THOSE WHO USE OUR SERVICES

At the centre of all work within health and care settings must be the needs of the people who use our services. All voluntary and statutory agencies would acknowledge this primary aim but may differ in how they view the recipient of their services. These differences manifest themselves in the term used to describe the recipients. Within health and social care settings a variety of terms have been used over time to describe the person being helped or supported. Currently, the term in vogue is 'service user', but it might still be 'patient' or 'client' in health/counselling settings. Lindon and Lindon (2000) chart the service traditions that have led to the use of different terms for service users in health and care settings. There is an ongoing debate as some people believe that the term 'service user' has negative connotations.

SUMMARY

In summary this chapter has established the following key learning points:

- Counselling skills are a set of tools that can be used in work and social settings to enhance helping relationships.

- Effective listening is at the core of helping relationships.
- Three important theoretical models to apply to helping relationships in health and social care settings are Carl Roger's core conditions, Gerard Egan's three-stage Model and John Heron's six-stage category intervention framework.
- The core counselling skills are reflecting, paraphrasing and summarising.

The next chapter explores using counselling skills in helping others.

Chapter 5

Using Counselling Skills to Help Others

Lindsey Neville

Key themes

This chapter explores

- the importance of counselling skills in the helping professions;

- recognising our own limitations;

- ethical dilemmas;

- referral;

- self-disclosure;

- transference;

- self-development.

This chapter builds on Chapter 4 and develops your knowledge about the use of counselling skills in the helping relationship. It explores the importance of counselling skills in the helping professions, the nature of helping relationships and the care of self within that process.

THE IMPORTANCE OF COUNSELLING SKILLS IN THE HELPING PROFESSIONS

The use of counselling skills has always been at the core of helping professions such as teaching, nursing, the police, social work and social care, but it is only in recent years that training for these professions has acknowledged its central role. When I trained as a teacher in the mid-1970s the curriculum contained no input on listening or counselling skills. There appeared to be an implicit understanding that those staff with an apparent aptitude for the work would naturally take it on board and absorb it into their workload. Colleagues with social care and health backgrounds tell me that this also reflects their experiences at the start of their careers. The changes that we have seen in recent years with regard to this recognition of the importance of counselling skills in the helping professions might be due to a number of different things.

- Changes in the nature of family life which mean that grown-up children may no longer be able to enjoy and utilise the support of their extended family and cultural groups because they live further away from these traditional sources of support.
- In 1982 there was recognition of positive messages from research about improved outcomes for service users when the Barclay Committee report (1982), a government prospectus for the planning of future social work, recognised the role that counselling skills might play in the future of social work. 'Counselling skills should be used in social work practice to help people tolerate the emotional impact of their world.'
- Acknowledgement from service users of the positive outcomes from interactions with professionals who use listening skills proficiently. I think that this means not just listening, but really concentrating on how someone says something.
- Patients, service users and carers identify good communication as one of the key attributes of a good nurse (Rush and Cook, 2006).

The nature of a helping relationship is that it is one into which each person enters by choice. At the heart of any helping relationship are respect, values and understanding, which we have explored in the previous chapter. In our modern society each one of us has our own set of values, which will determine the kind of helping relationships that we form with others. Some people will believe that individuals should be able to resolve their own issues without any external influences. Others will feel that some support might be helpful but potential help-seeking behaviour is perhaps hampered by old ideas that talking about something can only make it worse. Many readers may remember parents or grandparents telling them 'least said soonest mended', which suggests that difficult emotions are best resolved by keeping quiet about them. However, there will also be those who will have been told 'a problem shared is a problem halved'.

RECOGNISING OUR OWN LIMITATIONS

Individuals can choose whether or not they use counselling skills in their relationships with others. When you use counselling skills successfully people will find it easy to talk to you. This is likely to mean that service users will confide in you, telling you their stories and expressing painful emotions. Not only will our personal experiences and values affect the help that we give to others, but the issues that we discuss with service users will have an impact on our own wellbeing. In Chapter 4 I talked about the role of supervision for those who work as counsellors. This formal, professional support is rarely available for those who work within helping relationships using counselling skills. In many health and social care settings however, there will be support available from colleagues and/or line managers. Discussing your concerns with a colleague or line manager (within your confidentiality agreement) can be very helpful as they can offer you support, ease isolation and perhaps make suggestions that you may have overlooked.

It is important to remember that, when coping with the pain and distress of others, we are our own first priority. We cannot be a resource for others unless we take care of ourselves. We have a duty of care to ourselves as well as to others. Try not to underestimate the effect that helping people will have on you. It is likely that sharing the stories of others means that you will rarely hear their 'good news' but regularly hear their pain. Listening to the emotional pain of others may trigger your own emotional response. Therefore, those undertaking this kind of work need to think carefully about how they will manage these concerns. In thinking about this aspect of the work I want to encourage you, through this chapter, to adopt your own way of taking care of yourself. Each of us needs to take a personal stance as we all cope with things differently. However, there are some core coping strategies that I will identify and explore. I will also share my own personal mechanisms which others may find helpful.

Reflection

Pain can be understood as an expression of a social relationship. When we witness other people's pain, whether it is emotional or physical, suffering is given credence by our capacity to empathise with it.

(Orbach, 2004)

- Consider this statement and think of a situation when you have witnessed or experienced someone's distress.
- How did it make you feel?
- Did it change how you viewed the other person?

This might lead us to think that there are only negative consequences of hearing the distress of others. However, Orbach (2004) goes on to say that 'our capacity to register and endure it [the pain] of others enhances our experience of life'.

- How do you think your own life might be enhanced by listening to other people's pain?

It is important to be able to identify the point at which listening to other people has started to overwhelm you. I am fortunate to have shared my life for the last 30 years with my husband who can act as my 'barometer', by which I mean that he can tell me when I seem to be showing signs of stress that I may not have acknowledged. Perhaps there is someone in your life who could give you feedback on any changes that they might detect in your behaviour? I also recognise that when I become overwhelmed with aspects of my working life, I cut out doing those things which I enjoy and which help me relax and give balance to my life. I find it difficult to find time to go shopping with a friend, curl up on the sofa with a book or any number of other things that give depth, meaning and enjoyment to my life.

Research tells us that there are a number of other signs that might indicate to us that we are in danger of what many researchers call burnout (Skovholt, Grier and Hanson, 2001):

- spending less time with family and/or friends;
- withdrawing from other social activities that have previously given you pleasure;
- having difficulty sleeping;
- finding it difficult to make decisions;
- eating more or less than usual;
- finding it difficult to concentrate.

It is important to consider your own coping strategies. Research (Cartwright, 2003) shows that an effective way to manage the stresses of our working lives is to lead a balanced life. This can be achieved by having a wide circle of family and friends and a variety of interests. Achieving a good work/life balance is a challenge for us all and reflecting on your own balance is a good place to start in ensuring that you retain your own wellbeing.

Reflection

You can use the following website to enable you to reflect on whether your life is in balance and, if not, where the imbalance lies.
www.mindtools.com/pages/article/newHTE_94.htm

Developing personal coping strategies is important. Being empathic inevitably impacts on our own wellbeing because, as we have seen, it necessitates imagining that you are in the other person's shoes, which means that you are identifying very closely with their emotions. As I write this the media is full of stories about the missing four-year-old Madeleine McCann. There has been a national outpouring of concern for her and her family. People are imagining what it must be like to have a child go missing in such circumstances and it has created a very sombre mood among those who have been touched by the plight of both the child and the family. Speaking to friends, what happens is that they empathise with the family, but then the next step is to be thankful that it is not them; this begins the process of stepping back from the situation. This is a useful way of taking care of ourselves when we regularly hear distressing stories. It necessitates being clear in one's own mind that it is not our life and we are therefore slightly removed from the pain. It is a self-protection technique.

To ensure that I am regularly practising my skills in a formal setting, I see clients for the organisation RELATE. When I leave RELATE at the end of the evening my mind is often full of the work that I have done and the emotions of those whom I have worked with. I then need to begin a process of preparing to return to my everyday life, free of the clients' concerns. I achieve this in a number of ways:

- I concentrate on singing along with some of my favourite music on the way home.
- I compile a shopping list in my head for the next big supermarket shop.
- I make plans for the next weekend.
- I try to imagine my concerns and feelings for the client floating away from me down a river. This is called a visualisation technique and it can also be used for dealing with a variety of stressful situations. Some examples of how to use the technique can be found at the following website:

www.open.ac.uk/skillsforstudy/visualisation-for-dealing-with-stress.php

Reflection

When we use counselling skills in our work with others it is almost inevitable that they will express powerful emotions. This often means that they will cry. Think back to a time when you have cried about something.

- What did you feel like? What did those around you do?
- What would you have liked them to do?

There are a number of things that people do when someone cries. You might have thought of some of the following:

- Putting an arm round their shoulder.
- Giving them a hug.
- Holding or patting their hand.
- Giving them a tissue.

It is important to think about the effect of any response on the crying person. For example:

- this may be someone whom you barely know and therefore they might not welcome physical contact;
- culturally, physical contact may be inappropriate for some people;
- sometimes giving someone a tissue can be a thoughtful thing to do but do bear in mind that it can also send a message which says 'I am uncomfortable with you crying and so would like you to stop'.

The approach that you take will depend upon the nature of the relationship. If a friend of mine began to cry when she was talking to me, I would almost certainly hug her, but if someone I work with did the same I would just try to make sure that a box of tissues was in their field of vision and within their reach.

ETHICAL DILEMMAS

Each of us has our own set of standards or values that control how we behave. These will have been developed from a number of sources:

- parents;
- education;
- friends;
- work;
- experiences.

Reflection

Consider the following case study:
Mike has recently moved into a flat. He likes to use the internet but is struggling for money and doesn't think he can afford to pay for a connection. He discovers that there is a strong signal from a neighbour's wireless connection and decides to use it to access the internet.

- How do you feel about Mike's action?

Some people will feel that this amounts to theft and it is therefore unacceptable. Others will feel that it is doing no one any harm and is therefore acceptable.

- Have a discussion with friends about Mike's actions and you will be able to see the range of responses that it raises, though it is important to recognise that the law views Mike's action as dishonestly obtaining electronic communications services with intent to avoid payment, and it is therefore a crime.

Ethics are a code of conduct accepted by practitioners to ensure high standards in their professions. Different professions have different ethical frameworks. BACP's (2007) code of ethics informs the practice of its members and it applies to its members undertaking a variety of roles including providers of counselling skills. This framework places values, principles and personal moral qualities at the centre of professional practice. The code can also be seen as good practice for those who are not members but who still wish to adopt high standards in their practice. Other professions will have their own code of ethics, though the use of this term may vary in different settings and might be called a code of conduct, good practice guidelines or code of behaviour.

Reading activity

The ethical frameworks of the BASW and BACP are available for reading via the following websites:

British Association for Social Work **www.basw.co.uk/Default.aspx?tabid=64**

British Association for Counselling and Psychotherapy
www.bacp.co.uk/ ethical_framework/ethical_framework_web.pdf

- Have a look at these ethical frameworks and try to identify what they have in common.

When working with others there will be times when you experience an ethical dilemma. Professionally, an ethical dilemma or problem arises when something connected with your practice conflicts with the ethical framework which should inform that practice. Occasionally there will also be a conflict between your personal beliefs and those demanded by your setting.

Reading activity

Follow the link to read an example of an ethical dilemma written by a student nurse **www.nursing-standard.co.uk/students/sidwell.asp**

This case study highlights the conflicts that can occur between what is most appropriate for the service user and the demands of the organisation. Do you agree with the writer of the case study that Mary's treatment was inappropriate?

When this kind of conflict arises it is important to raise it with your supervisor or line manager.

Confidentiality

Most codes of ethics will include a commitment to confidentiality. Confidentiality is very important both within a service and in our relationships with service users. It means that we make an undertaking not to discuss what the service user tells us with anyone outside the setting. It is at the core of enabling the service user to feel safe and to place trust in the helper. This confidentiality is rarely absolute as it has to operate within the law. Some settings may also apply their own additional restrictions on the confidentiality offered. Key legislation includes:

- Children Act 1989;
- Terrorism Act 2000;
- Children Act 2004.

The restrictions on confidentiality in this legislation mean that practitioners cannot promise to keep secret anything which puts another person at risk. It's important to ensure that service users understand the boundaries of confidentiality that apply to the relationships that they develop within settings. Confidentiality usually applies to all workers within a setting rather than to individual workers. This means that information can be shared between practitioners. I think it is important that those who share personal information with me understand that I cannot promise to keep everything secret. So, when I first meet a counselling client or perhaps a student for whom I have some pastoral responsibility, I say something like: 'Normally everything that you tell me will remain between the two of us. In very rare circumstances it may be necessary for me to talk to someone else about what you tell me, but if this should happen I will always talk to you about it first'. This firmly sets the boundaries of the relationship between us and gives the other person the responsibility for choosing what they want to say.

Reflection

Let me give you a different kind of example from my own practice as a counsellor of the kind of situations that can arise. An 18-year-old client, who I had been seeing for some time, told me that he no longer wanted to live. He had worked out a very detailed and plausible plan to take his own life. I had no reason to doubt his intention to do exactly what he had planned. It is not against the law in this country to commit suicide and so I could have taken the view that it was his decision to make. However, I felt that he was making the decision at a time of huge upheaval and unhappiness in his life and that if he could continue his own efforts to resolve some of the issues and receive further support from relevant agencies then he could overcome his feelings that his life was not worth living.

The stance that I took meant that, in line with the agreement that we made at the beginning of our sessions, I needed to tell him that I felt that I had to break the confidentiality agreement between us. It was a very sad and difficult session during which I tried to encourage him to talk to his GP so that further appropriate support could be arranged. Sadly, he felt unable to do what I asked and so I told him that I would ring his GP to alert him to my concerns. There are dangers with this kind of approach:

- the client may take his own life before the GP manages to intervene;
- the client may find it difficult to trust me (or any other professional) in the future.

- What do you feel about my approach with this client?
- In my position would you have behaved differently?

This is a dilemma on which not all counsellors would agree. Some would believe that the client was entitled to take his own life if he so wished with no interference from anyone else.

REFERRAL

Referral is about recognising that you or your organisation might not be the most appropriate to help the person that you are talking to. We need to be able to recognise when another organisation or individual is better placed to offer support than ourselves. Although many statutory and voluntary organisations will have an extensive range of provision for service users, all practitioners and settings will have limitations.

An example of what it means to be referred, which many of us will have experienced, is when a referral is made by a GP. If a patient visits their GP with a health concern that the GP can't resolve, they expect the doctor to suggest that they consult another doctor who is a specialist in their condition. Referral needs to be handled sensitively as people might feel frightened or rejected. There are three important skills in referral:

1. Recognition of your own level of expertise.
2. Knowledge of other agencies.
3. Telling the other person that you are not the best person to help them.

Recognising your own level of expertise

It is important to recognise your own level of expertise. When we begin a helping relationship with someone it is almost impossible to know the kind of help that they might need. This is because their presenting problem may just be the top layer of a number of others. Think about people's potential difficulties as an onion. All you see at first is the top layer but underneath each layer will be another until you reach the core of the onion. Some people may want to talk about only the first layer; others may want to uncover more; some people will want to explore the very core. The top layer may be something that we are perfectly comfortable and trained to work with but the same might not be true of subsequent 'layers' – we won't know that until we have spent some time with the service user. In some cases it will be apparent as the first layer is uncovered that another agency or individual will be more appropriate and it will be necessary to tell the service user that someone else is better placed to help them. You will then need to identify who that person might be. Where the nature of the problem changes as the service user peels back the layers, you will need to assess, as new information becomes available, whether or not you are still the most appropriate helper. There are two ways to do this:

1. Regular personal reflection.
2. Discussion with a supervisor or line manager.

It's not only a valuable professional skill but also a useful life skill to have a good understanding of the range of statutory and voluntary agencies available to support service users. This understanding can then be used to identify appropriate sources of support so that service users can be directed appropriately. When I find myself in a position where I become aware that I am not the person best placed to help the person sitting with me, it is important to share that awareness with that person. There are specialist services that can offer a more appropriate service in certain circumstances. More information about making a referral and some of the available referral agencies can be found in Neville (2007).

Reflection

Consider where you might refer the following service users:

- a service user with a relationship issue;
- a service user whose words or actions seem bizarre to you;
- a service user who tells you that they think they have a problem with alcohol.

Telling the other person that you are not the best person to help them protects them and you from inappropriate interventions. If you have already helped the service user to peel back some of their layers, they will already have developed a relationship with you. If you have been effective in your active listening they will have grown to trust you and will value their relationship with you. If you manage this situation sensitively they will value your advice in seeking other help.

Imagine that you have just spent some time telling a practitioner about a distressing and difficult area of your life. The practitioner listens and then says, 'I can't help you, contact your GP/a counsellor/a social worker'.

- How would you feel?
- Can you think of other ways in which you might tell that person that you feel someone else might help them more appropriately?

It would be natural to feel rejected if, after trusting someone with your thoughts and feelings, they then move you down what might seem like a conveyor belt to other forms of help. That isn't to suggest that we should prolong relationships with service users if we don't have the skills to help and support them. Trying to help people when you are not equipped with the right tools can cause untold damage in the long run. However, referring people to other agencies and practitioners needs to be done very sensitively.

SELF-DISCLOSURE

If we are effective in establishing, in our relationships with service users, the core conditions that we explored in Chapter 4, it will sometimes be appropriate to offer some personal information about ourselves. This is called self-disclosure and it takes place when a helper is willing to share relevant and significant personal information with a service user. When shared appropriately this can be used to:

- encourage the service user to say what they want to;
- show them that they are not alone in their feelings and/or experiences;
- demonstrate your own humanity.

You should be aware that there are dangers here and I feel that it is better not to use self-disclosure at all than to over-use it. Where there is an over-sharing of personal information it can:

- take the emphasis away from the service user;
- create an impression of what I call 'been there, done that, got the t-shirt', which can undervalue the experiences of the service user.

Each one of us needs to decide what, if anything, we are willing to share from our personal lives. This can then be used in a controlled way to benefit the service user. For example, I often work with those who are struggling to come to terms with the death of someone that they loved. In this situation I find that individuals often find it helpful for me to tell them a little of my feelings and coping strategies following the death of my father. This seems to help in a number of ways:

- They can see that it is possible to endure the pain of bereavement.
- It can normalise the service user's own response to death.
- It can help them to feel that their pain is understood.
- It may help them project to a time when they too will be able to live life again.

TRANSFERENCE

Transference takes place when we transfer to others, feelings and attitudes that we once associated with important figures such as parents, teachers, etc. in our early life (see **www.cancerweb.ncl.ac.uk/cgi-bin/omd/feelings**). Let me give you an example of what I mean, from my own experience.

I once worked as a counsellor in a college of further education. I had a client whom I saw over many weeks. Lauren came to see me initially because she felt that her relationship was under pressure from her return to education. Her partner was struggling to accept the changes that had taken place and she felt that the relationship was finished. Over the months that I saw her I came to know her very well and we worked on what she wanted from the relationship and whether he was likely to be able to offer it to her. Her low self-esteem became apparent as we worked and I was aware that she responded to me in what I felt was a child-like way. As we worked together I realised that she had transferred her feelings and attitudes towards her mother on to me. She had begun to look to me to tell her what to do rather than to explore options with her. Her mother was someone who had commanded great authority and demanded obedience and had always told her daughter what to do. Lauren had transferred onto me her mother's attitudes, expecting me to behave and respond as her mother would have done.

Counter-transference happens the other way. So a helper will respond to the behaviour, feelings or attitudes of the client. To continue the same example, counter-transference would have occurred if I had begun to respond to Lauren as if I were her mother. You can read more about transference and counter-transference in a short article by Jackson (2004) which is listed in the References at the end of the book.

SELF-DEVELOPMENT

As helpers we can all build on our skills base to enhance the work that we do with service users. Undergraduate courses in health and social welfare usually include a Level 4 module on counselling skills, with perhaps a Level 5 development module on counselling theory and practice. However, these are sometimes optional rather than mandatory modules. These are also often modules that have a high level of emphasis on practical skills and will equip students with an understanding of the relevant issues. Those who wish to enhance their skills further might wish to take up one of the many counselling skills courses available through further education colleges and a range of private providers.

By following one of these shorter courses, some students may find that they have an aptitude and an enthusiasm for the work and may wish to progress to counsellor training. There is a number of agencies that offer further training opportunities.

- A BACP information leaflet (further details are available in the References section at the end of the book) gives details of relevant information for intending counsellors in England and Wales, and lists the courses available which will lead to accreditation by the BACP.
- COSCA (Counselling and Psychotherapy in Scotland) provides similar information for courses in Scotland.
- CPCAB (Counselling and Psychotherapy Central Awarding Body).
- OCR (Oxford Cambridge and Royal Society Arts Examinations).
- Voluntary agencies such as RELATE, Samaritans, CRUSE Bereavement Care, etc.

There are a variety of routes into counselling as a profession and those practising as counsellors have made very different journeys. In Reid (2004) a number of counsellors describe their journeys. The text also highlights the day-to-day lives of counsellors working across a variety of statutory and voluntary agencies and will give a helpful insight into the nature of the work.

This chapter has explored a range of issues relating to using counselling skills in helping others. It has provided a variety of resources for you to explore and learn from. In the final chapter we will explore putting all our communication and interpersonal skills into action.

Chapter 6

Communication and Interpersonal Skills in Practice

Elaine Donnelly

Key themes

This chapter builds on previous chapters and explores

- things that are important to people;
- the experience of care: a service user's perspective;
- using the skills of empathy, active listening and self awareness;
- working in organisations and communicating with others;
- the written word;
- the telephone and e.mail;
- face-to-face communication;
- dealing with difficult people.

THINGS THAT ARE IMPORTANT TO PEOPLE

As a student working, or hoping to work, in a health or social care setting you will find it useful to spend some time reflecting upon what it is like to be at the receiving end of the care that you and your organisation offer. This chapter will review what is important to you and others when considering care, and it makes use of a care study to illustrate an elderly person's perception of being admitted into care and the perception of his informal carers. Using the principles that are highlighted within that experience we will explore how to deal with difficult situations, how to diffuse emotional outbursts and how to approach communication with difficult people.

This final chapter seeks to use all the principles and details that have been discussed in previous chapters with regard to communication and interpersonal skills and therefore assumes that the reader is familiar with the same. To begin the work of Chapter 6 I would like to ask you what you think are the most important things in your life.

Reflection

- I would like you to think about all those things that are really important to you. They may be tangible things that you own or possess, or they may be abstract ideas or considerations that you hold to be of value to yourself and others. You might wish to take your time over this reflective activity, sharing your thoughts and ideas with those people close to you and perhaps extending that to the people you study and work with.

- Having reflected on those issues most dear to you, I would now like you to identify a list of 20 of the most important things to you in the world but, before you do that, I am going to impose some limits on what can be held in your list:

- family members are to be regarded as one choice;
- loved ones and friends are to be regarded as one choice;
- pets, regardless of their species and number, are also to be regarded as one choice.

That's three on your list, what are the other 17?

- Just in case you are struggling to put pen to paper, reflect on the following as this might just help focus your thinking.
  - What would you save in the event of a disaster such as a fire or a flood?
  - What would you/do you hide from potential thieves?
  - If you were taken into prison what would you want to safeguard?
  - If you were forced to live under a different political régime that is very different from that which you know, what would be most important to you?
  - Bad things happen to people all the time in our world. What if they were to happen to you?

Here's my list:

- Family – that includes the people I love most of all in the world.
- Friends – a life without friends would be empty.

- My happy box, which contains all sorts of daft-looking oddments and souvenirs but they are important to me.
- Photographs – there are many albums detailing different experiences and people in my life.
- My privacy – I hold it dear.
- My right to speak out and voice my opinion.
- My own space and the freedom to choose to be where I want to be.
- My books – I have many.
- My CD collection from ABBA to Zeppelin.
- My computer and all my memory sticks (that may count as two).
- My lovely car – it's not brilliant but it gets me about.
- Good food and wine – I do love both.
- My job and my role as a senior lecturer, and contact with students.
- My allotment and all the fruit and vegetables it produces.
- My mobile phone.
- The beautiful jewellery that people have bought me over the years.
- My independence.
- My knowledge of the world and my mental capacity (that's two really).
- Making my own decisions about how I live.
- My physical health.

Creating that list, knowing that it would be up for public view, was no easy task, even though I am experienced in helping others to do the same. Perhaps you struggled or maybe you found it easy. Does your list go beyond 20 items? Can you compare your list with other people's lists? Are they similar in any way?

My guess is that there are many things similar within our lists but, regardless of similarity or differences, the most important thing is that the list represents what is important to you and can be seen as a marker of who you are and what you hold dear. Our personality is often portrayed by the things we hold dear. (If you are interested in finding out a little about yourself and your personality you might wish to follow this link and take the adapted Myers-Briggs Personality Test **www.humanmetrics.com/cgi-win/ JTypes2.asp**)

Understanding ourselves and other people

Psychology can teach us a great deal about ourselves and about other people and, as a person working in the care services, it is important that you understand some of the basic tenets of psychological study. Understanding yourself and how you prefer to be with others will provide you with valuable information about your personal communication style and why you get on well with some people and not others. Adapting our responses to individuals can help the communication process to flow more easily.

Psychology can also be useful in helping us understand the impact our self-esteem has upon us as individuals and, in particular, the way in which self-esteem is important to psychological health. How we feel about ourselves and what we hold dear is directly affected by changes in our health status. Gross and Kinson (2007) discuss the development of the self concept and offer examples of how changes to our physical bodies can impact on our perception of self and consequently alter our behaviour. Indeed, the whole text is worthy of a read.

Reflection

I want you now to think about a person that you have had experience of working with or being with who has had to be admitted into care, health care as an emergency, or social care as a planned event as a consequence of alterations in their physical or psychological health.

- Using your skills of self awareness and empathy, imagine what it must have been like to be that person.
- What was the response from the care agencies involved?
- If you found yourself in a similar situation, how would you feel?

If you were that person and had that experience of being admitted into care, how many things on the list that you previously generated do you think would still be immediately available to you? Work systematically through your list of 20 things and score out those that would not be available. Then erase components of those things that perhaps may be available but only in small measures. For example, your family and friends whose access to you is likely to be limited due to visiting rules. You can't have all your photos with you but you could have a snapshot in your purse/wallet. It's all about compromise. On admission into care it is likely that you would be advised about the safe-keeping of valuables and you would be asked to turn off your mobile phone. It is more than likely that your privacy would be seriously invaded with questioning and possible examination and your right to be free to determine your own daily activities would be, in the first instance, severely curtailed. Your car would be left at home as parking is always expensive and difficult, and you certainly would not have your own bed or chair. Everything around you would be unfamiliar.

Go through your list and share your thoughts with a friend, fellow student or your teacher or mentor and see what is left on that list as a result of being admitted into care. It is likely that you will strike out the majority of those things you listed.

I always find this a sobering thing to do but it is a really useful exercise to undertake because it gives us an insight into what people experience when they are taken from their own surroundings, either because they are too ill or just too frail to take care of themselves. The admission into care is often not a positive experience.

The people who are in need of either health or social care lose so much in accepting the care that they need. The arguments as to whether it is 'for the best' fade in comparison with what a person has to give up in relation to their independence and freedom 'to be'. Nicholson-Perry and Burgess (2002) discuss the ways in which people who suffer serious illness have to adapt, both psychologically and socially, as their health status changes. With illness comes a personal change of perception of who we are, and our lifestyle and relationships all have to change too. When a person is faced with so much loss, the feelings of the Child ego state can be overwhelming. Despair, fear, anger, abandonment, grief, resentment and bitterness are, sadly, common experiences of those admitted into care.

Case study: an experience of care

The following case study is offered to help you understand what it can be like to be admitted into care and how important communication is throughout that process. This is just one person's story and the consent of the gentleman to whom this happened has been sought and agreed. Bill Jones, whose name has been changed to protect his identity, has read the chapter and confirms the content. Seeking consent is described by Bradshaw and Merriman (2007) as a 'fundamental part of a therapeutic relationship' and they comment that 'seeking consent is a process and not just a one-off event'. Bill hopes that his story will go some way to helping others see what it is like to be admitted into care and that it will help improve the communication skills of carers, particularly in those first few weeks that he described as being a particularly horrible time for him.

Bill is an elderly gentleman who has lived alone for many years following the death of his wife. He has no children but he was supported by good friends and neighbours who, over the years, took on many responsibilities to help ensure that Bill was safe and cared for. He was fiercely independent and had learned many new skills as he adjusted to living on his own but, as the years unfolded, his health deteriorated and arthritis took its toll on his mobility and his ability to care for himself. Like many elderly people he experienced several falls in the house and outside in his beloved garden, causing himself physical damage and resulting in him being fearful of being on his own. He had several emergency admissions to the local A&E department and, following a request for a social need assessment, arrangements were made for him to be supported at home. Several appliances were delivered to help with his daily activities – grab bars were situated around the house to help him mobilise and a commode was installed in his bedroom. He agreed to receive daily visits from a care agency who offered support with meals and help with personal and daily living activities. Although this meant Bill had to compromise on how he chose to live, he did adjust and the system worked reasonably well for some months.

Bradshaw and Merriman (2007) outline useful principles in communicating with the older person, paying particular regard to dignity, privacy and comfort. It would be true to say that all those people who served Bill in his own home were respectful of his personal space, paid regard to the normal protocols expected when entering someone's home and treated him as a fellow human being. There was a great deal of humour used by the workmen who fitted the grab bars and the delivery of the commode resulted in all the 'throne jokes' you can think of. This certainly helped to ease what was an uncomfortable situation for Bill. The skill of these people was to treat Bill as an equal and it worked. They all referred to him as Mr Jones and took no liberties in assuming the right to use his first name. The carers who came to the house soon established good rapport with him by being professional and respectful in helping him to meet his own needs. In your role as a carer it is extremely important to maintain that professional attitude towards those you work with, and you need to check all the time that your approach is acceptable to them. I am allowed to call Bill by his first name but I had known him for five years before he invited me to call him Bill. Friendship is not to be assumed, particularly when you are working as a professional, and calling older people by their first name without being invited to do so is often viewed by the older person as being forward and impolite.

Bill was determined to stay at home and the support system seemed to be working well but, while the neighbour who would normally call in at lunchtime was away on holiday, the late-afternoon carer arrived to find Bill on the floor where he had been for several hours, nursing a damaged forehead and a swollen wrist. He was in a poor condition, chilled to the bone, confused and unable to stand and, following a trip to the A&E department, he was admitted into residential care. It is reported that on admission into care he was confused, shouting loudly, demanding to be taken back home and was very rude to the people who tried to approach him. It was the ambulance driver who transferred Bill to the residential unit from the hospital who eventually calmed him down to the point that he agreed to stay at least for the time being.

This was a major life event for Bill to adjust to. What he deemed to be safe was not acceptable to the care service who had been invited in to help him at home. Bill was very angry that his independence was, as he describes it, 'being taken away from me'. He saw his life being taken apart and there was nothing that he could do to stop it. Had he the ability to walk, he would have walked away but he was almost immobile, bruised and battered from his fall and unable to cope alone. There was no family to rescue him and take him home, there was a lot of anger and resentment on his part and he blamed all the people around him for letting him down, even those who were trying to help. Bill was responding to what was happening to him from his Child ego state. He had all sorts of misconceptions about what happened to people when they were admitted into care and, as he said to me, 'I have never felt so helpless in all my life. I wanted to hit out at them but I couldn't even do that'.

Reading activity

We should stop here for a moment and consider the process of taking someone like Bill into care. There are several frameworks that offer guidance and advice in setting care standards for the elderly, in particular The National Service Framework for Older People (2001). This is available online at:
www.dh.gov.uk/en/publicationspolicyandguidance/dh_4003 066-17k

Another useful area to review is that of the Human Rights Act (1998). This is available online at **www.direct.gov.uk** You will find many useful links there to follow as you require. You may wish to supplement your reading with other texts in this series with regard to values and ethical dilemmas.

For those working with children and families I recommend a visit to the following website that will provide many links to legislative frameworks including the Children Act (2004) and other links concerning children and young people: **www.everychildmatters.gov.uk**

Taking anyone into any form of care is a major step, whether that care is planned or unplanned, scheduled or unscheduled, involves hospitalisation or any form of residential care. Consent must be sought whether the person is young or old and this can be achieved only by using good communication skills. Nicholson-Perry and Burgess (2002) comment that 'good communication empowers people to make informed choices that are right for them as individuals'. Sometimes those choices are limited as in the case of Bill who knew he had no alternative choices available to him at that time and had to accept the place that was found for him, albeit on a temporary basis. It was the responsibility of those around him to help him, to reassure him and to give him hope for the future. The way to do that is through good communication skills and proactively using coun-selling skills to help the person in crisis.

> Bill had an individual room at the end of a very long corridor, all very uniform in design, with lots of posters and information around detail-ing fire exits and directions to various locations. His room had an en-suite bathroom facility, his meals were ready cooked and served to him either within the dining room or in his own room, there was a doctor on call and care staff to assist him in everything he needed. It sounds idyllic but that is not how Bill saw it. When a friend visited she found he was dressed in someone else's pyjamas and his clothes were still in his suitcase. They had been left there because they were not labelled and there was a fear they would be lost. A congealed meal lay cold on a tray on his bed, which was too short for his tall frame, and he had only one pillow, which was too soft to support his aching neck. He had not been allowed to walk alone for fear of another fall and he had to rely on the staff attending to him for his every need. One of the young women carers even called him Mr Billy. He was not impressed. His complaints to his friend would fill many pages but all she could do at that point was to listen as his Child ego state poured out all the injustices to which he felt he had been subjected. He was angry, he was cross, he was scared about the future and he cried.

Dealing with anger

Bill's friend took a very rational approach to the complaints that she heard and, operating in her Adult ego state, she acted as his advocate. She asked many direct questions of those who were responsible for caring for him, taking care to raise his complaints and concerns in a rational enquiring manner. The majority of the responses to the questions asked appeared to be defensive and the nurses and carers alike were often very patronising, causing ill feeling and distrust. Thomas (2003) shows that the combination of time constraints and high workloads often leaves nurses feeling defen-sive and responding to complaints in a defensive manner. Thomas goes on to outline the way in which defensiveness can add to the already emotional situation and result in anger. Anger and emotional outbursts are common-place in care settings. Where else would you find such vulnerable people? It is no surprise that anger is the most common emotion expressed.

As people working in health and social care facilities it is important to appreciate the role of anger in everyday living. Rather than viewing it as something to be feared, you need to explore what underpins and motivates anger and identify the ways in which you can harness the energy spent through anger, and use that energy elsewhere. Anger serves a really important function in life. It helps us cope with stress and to express our feelings. Anger and the expression of anger is influenced by our coping strategies, and our feelings of being out of control and vulnerable are often expressed as anger, which is often directed at those around us. Whether those around us deserve that anger is another issue but, for now, we will accept that anger is a common reaction to difficult circumstances and that none of us is rational all of the time. Working in a helping capacity you need to develop a strategy for coping with the expression of highly charged emotions by those receiving care and also to cope with the emotions of the families who observe the care process and also feel helpless. We'll look at some strategies that may be helpful a little later in the chapter.

> Staff cited Bill's mild confusion to explain many of his complaints, which made him feel even angrier and led to many verbal outbursts. This resulted in staff finding him difficult to communicate with and therefore withdrawing from him. Over a period of time Bill's anger turned to helplessness and he became increasingly unhappy and uncommunicative, which was interpreted as a decline in his condition. Despite an attempt to improve relationships and get people communicating with one another it was eventually agreed that the placement was not suitable and Bill, with the support and help of his friends and neighbours, set about finding somewhere that he would be happy to spend the rest of his days.

This was a man whose life was being curtailed in a way that he found unacceptable. He felt as if he had been locked away, and the way of living in this particular establishment encroached upon all the things he held dear. His privacy, his independence, his comfort, his freedom were all affected by things that were out of his direct control, and his day was determined by other people, many of whom he had no relationship with at all even after several weeks of living there. The breakdown in communication was unfortunate and indicated a need for communication training among the staff. Jelphs (2006) discusses the way in which the very mention of communication skills to health care professionals causes raised eyebrows. She states that 'something as fundamental as communication is seen as a soft skill' and goes on to comment that 'communication is the skill that can possibly have the greatest impact on effective health care delivery'. Communication and counselling skills can be learned and used by all helpers to help prevent breakdown in care and facilitate a positive care experience.

A new care home was found and the experience of being admitted into the new establishment was very different. First and foremost Bill had a say in where it was he should go. He visited several places before he made his choice. The transfer was planned and he saw his room before accepting it to be his. He negotiated with care staff about what he could have brought from home and this included a writing bureau, many papers and files detailing important information regarding his finances and history, his own TV and video recorder, his own duvet, pillows and bedding, several pictures, photographs, ornaments and, most important, his electric buggy and his pipe. He was invited to complete a questionnaire about his life and daily living activities, an assessment of his ability to care for himself was undertaken with his permission and a temporary contract for care was agreed.

Bill thought this to be very important. He wanted to make sure the home suited his needs before finalising details and signing up for the long term. This process was accommodated easily with the managers of the care home, who agreed wholeheartedly that there should be a trial period before Bill had to make up his mind and take up permanent residence.

On his arrival at his new home Bill expressed many anxieties. What if he didn't like it, what about his house, what did he need to have immediately available to him, what about the cat, his newspapers and the mail, who would bring his things, etc? He was welcomed personally by the manager of the unit and his things were treated with great reverence and respect. Staff arranged to have all his clothes and bedding labelled and arrangements were made for the safe transportation of his possessions. His key worker sat with him and recorded all his concerns and then helped him map out strategies for dealing with all of them, contacting friends and neighbours on his behalf. Bill now has a new daily routine. He has a choice in meals and always eats at the table, apart from breakfast which he prefers in his own room. He has freedom of movement and his electric buggy has a parking place close to hand. He has a room with a door leading to the outside world where the gardens are splendid and he is free to roam during daytime hours. So he can go and smoke his pipe in the garden at peace. One of the carers supplied him with a bird guide book so that he could learn the names of the birds that visited the feeding table situated outside his window. He has a safety call button that he wears around his neck in case he is in need of urgent assistance, and he has at hand his own money and easy access to an expense account set up by his solicitor, who has Power of Attorney and is now overseeing his finances and the sale of his house.

There is a great deal of political debate about the payment of care bills in this country but I do not have room to discuss this here. The most important thing for Bill is that he had the opportunity to request the setting up of the legal process for Power of Attorney as he recognised that his confusion is likely to increase as he grows older. Coming to this point of self-awareness was all part of the change process for Bill. Many people helped him through those difficult decisions and realisations by having Adult to Adult ego state conversations with him, finally arranging for him to meet with his nominated solicitor. Just because someone has episodes of confusion does not mean that Adult to Adult conversations are impossible. Avoiding difficult conversations that need to be held only makes things worse in the long run. If you adhere to the Rogerian principles outlined in Chapters 3 and 4 you will get the best out of people and empower them to maintain a level of personal integrity.

Bill has commented that the difference between this unit and the first one is that the staff listen to him, pay him due regard and respect his wishes. If he needs more toothpaste it is collected, if his whiskey runs out he can arrange for a new bottle to be purchased for him. He can wander around the gardens in his buggy and smoke his pipe out of doors. He can invite friends to lunch with 24-hours notice and he has his own mobile phone with him to keep in contact with his friends when he chooses. There is a residents' committee with which he is involved and there are lots of activities that he can either observe or take part in. Bill is still frail and at times confused and very cantankerous but he accepts that he needs care and accepts the care on offer. The staff in this unit demonstrate a positive regard towards him. The overarching philosophy of this unit is that it is the person's home and it should be as comfortable as their previous home was. Everything is achievable with a little thought and application and the staff use the skills of empathy and show the ability to understand what it is like to be old and frail and in Bill's situation. They actively listen to him and communicate with him in a positive way. He has become a person again.

USING THE SKILLS OF EMPATHY, ACTIVE LISTENING AND SELF-AWARENESS

When communicating with people who use your services it is really important to try to step into their shoes and experience the world as it is for them. The qualities of holding people with unconditional positive regard, demonstrating congruence in your behaviour and words, being warm and genuine and using empathetic responding skills is the mark of a good communicator and someone whom people will feel comfortable with. Being on the 'other person's side' will enable you to communicate more effectively with the people in your care. Good communication can really help even the most vulnerable people to make informed choices and decisions about what is to happen to them.

Bonham (2004) introduces the student to communicating as a mental health carer and comments that we should never underestimate the potential for helping others simply by listening to them. Bonham goes on to discuss the process of thoughtful communication in a caring relationship exploring intuition, the concept of ordinariness, being optimistic and the myth of the magic sentence. He concludes that 'the process of helping people can be a long and relentless process that takes time and input from many different professionals'. This is illustrated by Bill's experience. There were times when the process was so slow and communications with various professions were often held up causing untold frustration. Even though he is now happily placed in a care home that meets his current needs, no one can say that things will not change, so the process must continue.

Individuals are ultimately responsible for their own input, and developing the skills of self-awareness is the first step to the development of good communication and interpersonal skills. Exploring those intra-personal aspects of the self as discussed in Chapter 1 can be facilitated through the use of the communications theory of Transactional Analysis as detailed in Chapter 3. We need to know and understand our own self, what Myers Briggs calls our 'preferred way of being'. We need to be able to view ourselves from other people's perspectives and, to be a good communicator, we need to embrace a philosophy of care that holds at its core the ideals of humanity and wholeness. Seek feedback from others, undertake training when it is available and read as much as you can. Jelphs (2006) details how health care professionals need to be open to other people and their considerations and perceptions, and suggests that listening and observing tape recordings of ourselves provides an ideal opportunity to see ourselves as others see us.

WORKING IN ORGANISATIONS AND COMMUNICATING WITH OTHERS

Just as we need to listen to ourselves, those in our care and those who can give us feedback about our performance, we also need to listen to those with whom we work in partnership. Carnwell and Buchanan (2005) make clear the point that in recognising the needs of those we care for we must also recognise the role of others in providing for people's needs. There is a danger within service provision to see only that which we can offer and ignore what other agencies and professionals can provide. Effective care relies on us being able to work in partnership, and being able to communicate with people from other agencies ensures that those we care for receive the best possible care.

Carnwell and Buchanan (2005) outline the dangers of professional groups working in isolation. Specialisation and professionalism have led us to a situation where subject-specific language can be difficult to understand and often contributes to a breakdown in communication between agencies and organisations. It is recognised that understanding the role of others will help in ensuring seamless working with people. Networking and joined-up thinking are now at the centre of providing effective care, and professional and volunteer groups need to find new ways of communicating and working in partnership. Jelphs (2006) outlines what she believes to be the key areas for organisations, teams and individuals to consider.

- How to develop and implement a meaningful communication strategy.
- How the strategy links to other strategic policies and procedures.
- How information is shared between staff.
- The ability of staff to access communication systems.
- How information is shared between patients and service users.
- How to develop information that is empowering and enabling for staff and service users.
- How to manage the grapevine.
- How to manage the media.

These are all big issues to consider. Sharing information requires a language that all can understand and developing that level of understanding requires everyone involved to be proactive and open to change. Carnwell and Buchanan's (2005) *Effective Practice in Health and Social Care* is a useful text to help you understand some of the challenges that the caring services currently face and is well worth a read.

CODES OF PRACTICE

As previously discussed, poor communication is often at the centre of complaints that people make against the NHS, and staff attitude in particular is one of the main reasons for complaint. The NHS is a massive organisation and the communication systems are many, with each one tailored to meet the need for recording and sharing information. The NHS Records Management Code of Practice is available online at **www.dh. gov.uk/enPolicyandguidance/organisationalpolicy/Records management/ index.htm** This website provides a great deal of material to read with regard to communication, and the links there are very useful covering all aspects of modes and channels of communication that were discussed in

Chapters 1 and 2. Organisations that seek to help people must have criteria that they use to guide the practice of those who work for them. Codes of practice offer criteria that can be used to review your own personal performance as a person working in the helping professions and may also be used by your employers to judge your practice and your ability.

> ## Reflection
>
> Which code of practice do you use to review your performance? The following websites are recommended to you, subject to your specific role: **www.nmc-uk.org** for nurses and midwives and the General Social Care Council (GSCC) codes of conduct are available at: **www.gscc.org.uk/ Good+practice+and+conduct/Get+copies+of+our+codes/**

OTHER MODES OF COMMUNICATION

The written word

Each of these codes of conduct makes reference to communication and record-keeping. Working with people will require you to take part in recording detail. Being able to maintain clear and accurate records will be part of your role. The level of supervision that you receive will be subject to your role and position within the organisation but there may come a time when you are responsible for writing and maintaining official records.

In an increasingly litigious society it is of great importance that the records we keep are meticulous. They are an important means of communication between staff and agencies and are available to the individual at their request. Records were previously kept mainly in paper form but, with the development of technology, they are increasingly being kept in electronic form. It is important to remember that the contents and quality of these records will have consequences for those being cared for and for you as the carer. They are legal documents that may be called for scrutiny at any time. As such, records should be:

- accurate in their detail;
- contemporaneous (meaning up-to-date);
- non-judgemental - there is no room for subjective material;
- legible, others must be able to read them;
- kept safe and maintain confidentiality.

The Data Protection Act (1998) is available online at **www.england-legislation.hmso.gov.uk.acts/acts1998** and details the legal principles that underpin the regulation of the processing of information relating to people. You should familiarise yourself with these details to protect yourself and the people whom you work with.

The telephone

How many times have you tried to communicate with an organisation via the telephone and been left feeling really frustrated? You may recall from Chapter 2 that only 7 per cent of the communication that takes place normally is via the words used, so it is no wonder that the telephone is so difficult to use and so fraught with problems. If you look back to the discussion regarding communication models, the Transmission Model was designed specifically to help overcome difficulties experienced in telecommunication. Many organisations now give training on customer care and telephone technique and this has come about as a response to the many complaints received. It is important that you seek the advice and training of your employer but the following principles will certainly help you avoid running into difficulty when answering the phone.

- Clearly state the name of the organisation/agency or place of work.
- State your name and your position.
- Ask how you can help, for example:
    - Ward 10 Redwood hospital, Susan Jones, student nurse, can I help you? or…
    - Ashleigh Wood Care Home, Gillian Smith, receptionist, can I help? or…
    - Northwood Rehabilitation Unit, Tom Brown, care assistant, can I help?

You need to find the most comfortable way of introducing yourself, your status and your place of work. You may wish to say 'hello' or 'good afternoon' and that preference is up to you but the principle here is that when a person calls they need to know they have the right telephone number and to whom they are speaking. A good reply is one that gives those details, one that sounds professional and calm and one that is welcoming of the telephone call. If you have stated those things clearly it is likely that the caller will then respond positively, i.e. 'Yes, this is Doctor Mead, can I speak to …'

Please don't just say 'hello' as it leaves the caller struggling as to what to say next and it is unprofessional. Even if you have access to a telephone that gives you the caller's identity, never assume it is them as other people may be using their phone. Also be aware that detail should not be given over the phone that is confidential. If in doubt, seek advice from your mentor or manager.

E.mail

The facility to send documents and communications via e.mail is a fantastic communication system. It saves time, it is auditable and it can be incredibly effective, but it is also one of the most frustrating, mainly because of the number of unnecessary e.mails that are sent. Round robins and circulars may raise the odd smile but they clutter up your in-tray and distract the eye from what may be important, and it is more than likely that your organisation would frown upon the system being used in such a way. Don't use the e.mail for anything it is not intended to be used for. Check your employer's policies for e.mail use and do not fall foul of it as your job could be at stake.

There are certain principles that you should be aware of when using e.mail and attending to the following will help to prevent misinterpretation and keep the message reasonably intact.

- Is e.mail the best mode of communication to use?
- Should you be sending this detail via e.mail and is it confidential?
- To whom are you sending it and what do you want them to do with it?
- If you are using your employer's computer system you must attend to their protocols.
- Address the e-mail carefully.
- Flag up if you want a reply, receipt or confirmation of reading.
- Be polite and use 'please' and 'thank you' as appropriate.
- Check the tone of the message.
- Try to be as concise and professional as you can.
- NEVER USE UPPERCASE, AS IT LOOKS AS IF YOU ARE SHOUTING.
- Check the spelling and the grammar before sending the e.mail.
- Send it only to the people who need to receive it.

The ease of sending messages via e.mail makes it an attractive option but remember that when messages are sent and received electronically you do not have that opportunity to talk face-to-face with that person and there is a danger that priorities will be missed and information misinterpreted. You will not be able to see the receiver's reaction nor judge how the e.mail was received. The very essence of e.mail suggests that a quick response is required. It is important that you take your time in wording the e.mail and detailing the response time to the receiver. Short turnaround times may result in quick decisions that have not been fully thought through.

Face-to-face

As previously stated, most of your contact when working with people will be face-to-face. People who require the helping services are likely to be vulnerable and experiencing a variety of emotions. The following points serve as a reminder of previous material provided in this book.

- Remember that you are the helper so be calm and professional at all times.
- Stay in your Adult ego state while offering nurture and reassurance.
- If possible, attend to the environment and keep things calm and private.
- Introduce yourself and ask the person how you should refer to them.
- Pay attention to body language and what it is saying to the other person.
- Remember SOLER – Sit Open Lean Eye contact Relax (Egan, 1998).
- Use paralanguage to confirm active listening and consider the tone of your voice.
- Assess and take into account possible communication difficulties.
- Consider using additional methods such as signage, pictures, etc.
- Ensure that you listen attentively and check that what you heard is correct.
- Sit square with an open posture. Lean forward and gain eye contact.
- Use appropriate language according to age, culture and gender.

Using these basic communication skills should serve you well for most superficial relationships but it is likely that you will be working in an environment where developing your use of counselling skills will enable you to perform your role in a much more meaningful and helpful way. Practising counselling skills really does help you to develop the skill that you already have. Remember the Rogerian principles of

- unconditional positive regard – accept the other person for who they are and avoid being judgemental about them;
- warmth and genuineness – be approachable and open to others and try to be congruent in your thoughts and actions;
- empathy – try to put yourself in their shoes and consider what it must be like for them. You are familiar with this situation – it is likely that they are not.

All these qualities can be developed via experiential learning techniques and the process of reflection. Burnard (2006) comes highly recommended if you wish to try out further experiential learning. Remember Gerard Egan's helping skills:

- Let the person tell their story as it is seen by them.
- Help them explore their options.
- Get them to try out their options and evaluate them.

When working with people it is important to remember what your intention is. You can use John Heron's six-stage Category Intervention Analysis to keep you focused.

- Informative – to give new information and inform the other person.
- Prescriptive – to offer advice and make suggestions.
- Confronting – to challenge previously-held ideas and help the person explore their options.
- Cathartic – to help the person express their emotions through tears or anger.
- Catalytic – to draw out other detail and to encourage reflection.
- Supportive – to reassure the other person and give hope confirming the other person's worth.

Good communication is described by Burnard (2006) as the bedrock of good care but sometimes even good communication and interpersonal skills cannot easily manage the situation, particularly when emotions are high. People are not rational all of the time. When faced by fear and uncertainty they respond angrily and this can create difficult situations which if not diffused adequately can lead to aggressive action.

DEALING WITH DIFFICULT PEOPLE

Reading activity

Difficult people are all around us. The category of difficult people may even include you! The Institute of Management Excellence has an online newsletter available at **www.itstime.com/mar99.htm** This website offers some really interesting links and explores how to deal with difficult people in the workplace through the use of Personality Dragons. The dragons include:

- greed;
- impatience;
- arrogance;
- stubbornness;
- self-deprecation;
- martyrdom;
- self-determination.

These are interesting takes on the different sorts of personalities that we find ourselves working with and the website offers tried-and-tested solutions for given sets of circumstances. The Institute of Management Excellence offers some very sensible advice about how to manage emotionally-fuelled conflict and in summary suggests the following.

- Question your own defensiveness. Why are you upset by this situation? Remember defensiveness often fuels anger, leading to a worse situation.
- Stay focused in an irrational attack. See it as a gift that you do not have to accept. It is not personal.
- Calmly ask the person what they are upset about and accept that there is some kernel of truth in their complaint.
- Ask for feedback – 'It sounds as if you have been misinformed, is this true?' Being on their side will enable you to diffuse the situation more quickly.
- Don't try to win the fight – it is best to go for a win-win situation.
- Listen carefully and ask questions to elicit the nature of the complaint.
- Appreciate and don't blame.

Conflict is seen as a mutual problem that needs to be dealt with, and understanding what motivates people and fuels their emotions will help to pull the situation back to something that can be agreed upon and worked on jointly. In circumstances such as these using leverage is a good strategy. For example, 'If you agree to come with me now I'll sort out an appointment with your social worker and we'll see if we can sort something out'.

Reflection

Sometimes people's anger can present you with specific problems. The *British Medical Journal* (BMJ) featured an editorial article on 24 April 1999 looking at the ethical dilemmas health care workers met when trying to care for a racist patient within a clinical setting. The patient mistakenly thought the junior house doctor was a racist too as she carried a copy of the BNF in her pocket. That's the British National Formulary indexing drugs and medications but the patient assumed that BNF stood for the British National Front. You can access the article at **www.bmj.com** and there follows a series of comments from a variety of health care workers who have found themselves in similar situations. Have a read and make up your own mind as to what you think you would do in that situation using your Code of Conduct as a guide for practice.

If your strategies for dealing with difficult people fail it is important to remember that even if other people do not behave or respond differently, you can. Self-awareness and a willingness to learn are essential requirements to developing your own skill but when the situation involves strong emotions in the people whom you are caring for or working with effective communication and interpersonal skills are crucial.

The most important thing for you to remember is to seek help if you find you are out of your depth. There are no medals available for people who attempt to deal with situations that they cannot handle and the rule of thumb is that if the situation scares you tell the person that you can't deal with that situation and that you have to leave to get someone else to help them. Most people when angry are operating from their Child ego state and are out of control. Being faced by someone who tells them that they cannot handle this situation is often enough to jolt them back to a temporary thinking state as they realise the impact they are having on other people.

In Figure 9 the Angry Child ego state on the left is verbally abusing the helper's Child ego state on the right. This other person's angry Child ego state is fuelled to some extent internally via the person's Parent ego state. The Critical Parent is conveying messages such as 'how dare they do this to me, I don't need to tolerate this, tell them just what you think of them right now.' The Adult ego state is not currently being accessed so there is very little thinking taking place.

Although the helper's Child ego state is naturally ready to respond to this person's anger by being defensive or by being angry back, they do not have to accept this interaction. They can instead choose to use rationality and respond from their Adult ego state, pitching to transact with the Adult ego state of the other person.

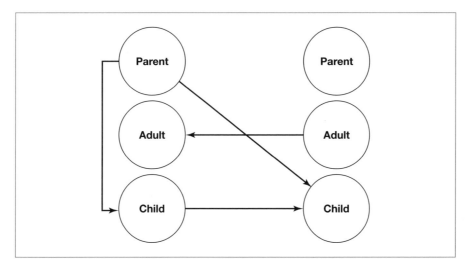

Figure 9 Transactional Analysis of dealing with a difficult person

For example, a safe Adult ego state response could be, 'you seem to be very upset and you do have a serious complaint to make but I am not really equipped to deal with this. Can you please wait here and I will get someone who can help you'. The other person's Adult ego state is being addressed in this transaction, resulting in a momentary diffusion of the situation and the Critical Parent ego state then needs to think and respond, probably with something like, 'yes, I do have a serious complaint to make, you had better go get somebody who can sort it out'. This will give you sufficient time to move away and seek help.

Genuine anger bursts out and results in tears as the emotion is burned out. The skilled communicator can stay with that person until the tears come and the emotional response begins to calm down. Those who stay angry are likely to be psychologically disturbed and pose a risk for others, and steps to safeguard others may need to be taken.

In the average working day it is likely that you will come across someone who is upset and my final bit of advice is never underestimate the power of a cup of tea. Challem (2007) outlines the effect of Theanine in tea, which is known to have a calming effect on people. For me the distraction of having to accept a cup of tea and co-ordinate holding the cup and drinking from it gives an upset person something to focus on. It enables thinking and as soon as people start to think about things again they are operating from the Adult ego state and it is then easier for them to control their emotion.

We all need to reflect on our own communication and interpersonal skills as they are fundamental to being an effective practitioner in whatever field you choose to work in. I trust that you have enjoyed reading and working with this text and I wish you well in your studies.

References

BOOKS AND JOURNAL ARTICLES

Abramowitz, J.S. (2001) 'CBT for Obsessive Compulsive Disorder; A Review of the Treatment Literature'. *Research and Social Work Practice*, 11(3), pp. 357–73

BACP (2006) *Choosing a Counsellor*. Rugby: BACP

Barclay Committee (1982) *Social Workers: Their role and tasks*. Bedford: Square Press

Beck, A.T. (1989) *Cognitive Therapy and the Emotional Disorders*. London: Penguin Press

Berne, E. (1957) *A Layman's Guide to Psychiatry and Psychoanalysis*. New York: Random House

Berne, E. (1961) *Transactional Analysis in Psychotherapy*. New York: Grove Press

Berne, E. (1968) *Games People Play. The Psychology of Relationships*. New York: Penguin Books

Berne, E. (1972) *What Do You Say After You Say Hello?* New York: Corgi Press

Berne, E. (1973) *Sex in Human Loving*. New York: Penguin Press

Berne, E. (1977) *Intuitions and Ego States. The Origins of Transactional Analysis. A series of papers*. San Francisco: TA Press

Blake, R. and Moulton, J. (1972) *The Diagnosis and Development Matrix*. Houston: Scientific Methods

Bonham, P. (2004) *Communication as a Mental Health Carer*. Cheltenham: Nelson Thornes

Bowlby, J. (1969) *Attachment*. New York: Basic Books

Bradshaw, A. and Merriman, C. (2007) *Caring for the Older Person*. Somerset: Wiley

Burnard, P. (1989) *Teaching Interpersonal Skills. A handbook of experiential learning for health professsionals*. London: Chapman and Hall

Burnard, P. (2006) *Counselling Skills for Health Professionals*. Cheltenham: Nelson Thornes

Carnwell, R. and Buchanan, J. (eds) (2005) *Effective Practice in Health and Social Care*. Milton Keynes: Open University Press

Cartwright, S. (2003) 'Work and Mental Health: An Employers' Guide D.M. Miller, M. Lipsedge and P. Lichfield (eds), Gaskell and Faculty of Occupational Medicine, London, 2002. *Stress and Health*, 19(2), p. 61

Cauchon, C. (1994) 'Talking to Oneself'. *Psychology Today*. Shropshire, England: Sussex Publishers

Crowley, P. and Hunter, J. (2005) 'Putting the public back into public health'. *Journal of Epidemiology and Community Health*, 59, pp. 265–7

Challem, J. (2007) 'Theanine. The Calm in your Tea'. *Better Nutrition*, 69(6) 32, pp. 34–5

De Board, R. (1998) *Counselling for Toads: A Psychological Adventure*. London: Routledge

Department of Health (2001) *Treatment choice in psychological therapies and counselling: Evidence based clinical practice guidelines*. London: Stationery Office

Department of Health (2007) *Trust, Assurance and Safety – The regulation of Health Care Professionals in the 21st Century*. London: Stationery Office

Egan, G. (1998) *The Skilled Helper*. Chichester: Wiley

Geldard, D. and Geldard, K. (2003) *Counselling Skills in Everyday Life*. Basingstoke: Palgrave

Gladwell, M. (2005) *Blink. The Power of Thinking without Thinking*. Washington: Time Warner Books

Goleman, D. (1996) *Emotional Intelligence. Why It Can Matter More Than IQ*. London: Bloomsbury

Grahame, K. (1908) *The Wind in the Willows,* London: Methuen

Gross, R. and Kinson, N. (2007) *Psychology for Nurses and Allied Health Professionals*. London: Hodder Arnold

Hargie, O. (ed.) (1991) *A Handbook of Communication Skills*. London: Routledge

Harris, T. (1969) *I'm OK, You're OK*. London: Pan Books

Harris, T. (1985) *Staying OK*. London: Pan Books

Heron, J. (2003) *Helping the Client* 5th Ed. London: Sage

Jasper, M. (2003) *Beginning Reflective Practice*. Cheltenham: Nelson Thornes

Jelphs, K. (2006) 'Communication: soft skill, hard impact?' *Clinician in Management*, 14, pp. 33–7

Johns, C. (2004) *Becoming a Reflective Practitioner* 2nd Ed. Oxford: Blackwell

Klein, M. (1980) *Lives People Live. A Textbook of Transactional Analysis*. Somerset, England: Wiley Press

Lambert, M.J. (ed.) (2003) *Bergen and Lambert's Handbook of Psychotherapy and Behaviour Change* 5th Ed. Chichester: Wiley

Lindon, J. and Lindon, L. (2000) *Mastering Counselling Skills*. Basingstoke: Palgrave

Littlejohn, S.W. and Foss, K.A. (2005) *Theories of Human Communication*. Belmont: Wadsworth/Thomson Learning

McLeod, J. (2001) *Counselling in the Workplace; the Facts. A systematic review of the research evidence*. Rugby: BACP

Neville, L. (2007) *The Personal Tutor's Handbook*. Basingstoke: Palgrave Macmillan

Nicholson-Perry, K. and Burgess, M. (2002) *Communication in Cancer Care*. Oxford: BPS Blackwell

Piaget, J. (1977) *The Essential Piaget*, H.E. Gruber and J.J.V. Gruber (eds). New York: Basic Books

Reid, M. (2004) *Counselling in Different Settings: The Reality of Practice*. Basingstoke: Palgrave

Rogers, C. (2002) *Client Centred Therapy*. London: Constable

Rogers, C.R. (ed.) (1967) *The therapeutic relationship and its impact; a study of psychotherapy with schizophrenia*. Madison: University of Wisconsin Press

Rush, B. and Cook, J. (2006) 'What Makes a Good Nurse? Views of Patients and Carers. *British Journal of Nursing*, 15(7), 14 April, pp. 482–5

Shannon, C. and Weaver, W. (1949) *The Mathematical Theory of Communication*. Urbana: University of Illinois Press

Skovholt, T., Grier, T. and Hanson, M. (2001) 'Career Counselling for Longevity: Self Care and Burnout Prevention Strategies for Counsellor Resilience'. *Journal of Career Development*, 27(4), pp. 167–76

Taylor, J. (2003) 'Managing staff development for online education: A situated learning model'. *Journal of Higher Education Policy and Management*, 25(1), pp. 75–87

Thomas, S.P. (2003) 'Anger. The Mismanaged Emotion'. *Dermatological Nursing*, 15(4), pp. 351–8

Trevethick, P. (2000) *Social Work Skills: A Practice Handbook*. Buckingham: Open University Press

West, R. and Turner, L.H. (2007) *Introducing Communication Theory: Analysis and Application*. New York: McGraw-Hill

Whitton, E. (1993) *What is Transactional Analysis? A Personal and Practical Guide*. Essex, England: Gale Centre Publications

Wood, J. (2004) *Communication Theories in Action: An Introduction*. Belmont: Wadsworth/Thomson Learning

WEBSITES

BACP (2005) Training and Careers in Counselling and Psychotherapy: **www.bacp.co.uk/education/T1.html** (accessed 1 May 2007)

BACP (2007) Ethics for Counselling and Psychotherapy: **www.bacp.co.uk/ethical_framework/** (accessed 8 March 2008)

BBC News (2007): **www.bbc.co.uk**

British Association for Social Work (2002) The Code of Ethics for Social Work: **www.basw.co.uk/Default.aspx?tabid=64** (accessed 16 May 2007)

Cambridge Learners Dictionary (2007): **www.cambridge.org/elt/dictionaries /cld.html** (accessed 9 May 2007)

Children Act (2004) and other links concerning childen and young people **www.everychildmatters.gov.uk**

Counselling and Psychotherapy in Scotland: **www.cosca.org.uk**

Counselling and Psychotherapy Central Awarding Body: **www.cpcab.org.uk**

Data Protection Act (1998) London: Stationery Office, HMSO: **www.england-legislation.hmso.gov.uk/acts/acts1998**

General Social Care Council (GSCC): **www.gscc.org.uk**

Jackson, K. (2004) Counselling Transference/Counter Transference Issues: **www.contactpoint.ca/bulletins/vb-n4.html** (accessed 2 May 2007)

Mindtools (2006) The Wheel of Life: **www.mindtools.com/pages/article/ newHTE_94.htm** (accessed 15 May 2007)

Myers Briggs Personality Test: **www.humanmetrics.com/cgi-win/JTypes2.asp**

National Audit Office (2006) Current Thinking on Managing Attendance: **www.nao.org.uk//publications/nau_reports/04-05/04051B_research paper.pdf**

Nursing Standard (2007) An Ethical Dilemma: **www.nursing-standard.co.uk/students/sidwell.asp** (accessed 25 May 2007)

Open University (2007) Visualisation Techniques for Dealing with Stress: **www.open.ac.uk/skillsforstudy/visualisation-for-dealing-with-stress.php** (accessed 7 June 2007)

Orbach, S. (2004) Everybody Hurts: **www.newstatesman.com/200402240044** (accessed 15 May 2007)

Oxford Cambridge and Royal Society Arts Examinations: **www.ocr.org.uk/**

Patient Advice Liaison Service: **www.dh.gov.uk//PatientAndPublicinvolvement/Patientadviceandliaison services/index.htm**

The Human Rights Act (1998): **www.direct.gov.uk**

The National Service Framework for Older People (2001): **www.dh.gov.uk/en/publicationspolicyandguidance/dh4003066-17k**

The NHS Records Management Code of Practice: **www.dh.gov.uk/enPolicyandguidance/organisationalpolicy/Records management/index.htm**

The Nursing and Midwifery Code of Conduct (2004): **www.nmc-uk.org**

Index